BUILDING
AND
SUSTAINING
A HOSPITAL-BASED NURSING
RESEARCH PROGRAM

Nancy M. Albert, PhD, CCNS, CCRN, NE-BC, FAHA, FCCM, FAAN, is the associate chief nursing officer of the Office of Research and Innovation, Nursing Institute, Cleveland Clinic Health System, Cleveland, Ohio, and a clinical nurse specialist at the Kaufman Center for Heart Failure, Cleveland Clinic, Cleveland, Ohio. She is also an adjunct associate professor at Case Western Reserve University, Bolton School of Nursing, Cleveland, Ohio, and a full professor at Aalborg University, Aalborg, Denmark.

As associate chief nursing officer of the Office of Research and Innovation, Dr. Albert administers and provides services throughout the Cleveland Clinic Health System, conducts her own program of research, and mentors nurses in research and evidence-based practice. Dr. Albert is also an external consultant and educator to nurses and health care teams wishing to promote evidence-based nursing practices, nursing research, and nursing innovations. Dr. Albert was given the Nurse of the Year award from the Greater Cleveland Center for Health Affairs (2000); the Partners in Research award from the Center for Hospice, Palliative Care and End of Life Studies, University of South Florida (2006); and the first annual Researcher of the Year award from the National Association of Clinical Nurse Specialists (2007). She was named the Distinguished Research Lecturer by the American Association of Critical-Care Nurses in 2013, and received the Cleveland Clinic Nursing Institute Lifetime Achievement Award in 2014. In October 2015, Dr. Albert was inducted into the American Academy of Nurses as a fellow. Dr. Albert has published over 230 peer-reviewed articles in nursing and medical journals, written book chapters, and presented nationally and internationally. She is the first past president of the American Association of Heart Failure Nurses, and volunteers on national committees for multiple medical, nursing, and health care organizations.

BUILDING
AND
SUSTAINING
A HOSPITAL-BASED NURSING
RESEARCH PROGRAM

Nancy M. Albert, PhD, CCNS, CCRN, NE-BC, FAHA, FCCM, FAAN

Editor

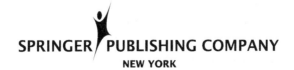

SPRINGER PUBLISHING COMPANY
NEW YORK

Springer Publishing Company, LLC
11 West 42nd Street
New York, NY 10036
www.springerpub.com

Acquisitions Editor: Joseph Morita
Production Editor: Kris Parrish
Composition: Westchester Publishing Services

ISBN: 978-0-8261-2814-0
e-book ISBN: 978-0-8261-2815-7

15 16 17 18 / 5 4 3 2 1

The author and the publisher of this Work have made every effort to use sources believed to be reliable to provide information that is accurate and compatible with the standards generally accepted at the time of publication. Because medical science is continually advancing, our knowledge base continues to expand. Therefore, as new information becomes available, changes in procedures become necessary. We recommend that the reader always consult current research and specific institutional policies before performing any clinical procedure. The author and publisher shall not be liable for any special, consequential, or exemplary damages resulting, in whole or in part, from the readers' use of, or reliance on, the information contained in this book . The publisher has no responsibility for the persistence or accuracy of URLs for external or third-party Internet websites referred to in this publication and does not guarantee that any content on such websites is, or will remain, accurate or appropriate.

Library of Congress Cataloging-in-Publication Data

Building and sustaining a hospital-based nursing research program / Nancy M. Albert, editor.
    p. ; cm.
    Includes bibliographical references and index.
    ISBN 978-0-8261-2814-0 (hardcopy : alk. paper) — ISBN 978-0-8261-2815-7 (ebook)
    I. Albert, Nancy M., editor.
    [DNLM: 1. Clinical Nursing Research—organization & administration.   2. Program Development—methods.   3. Nursing Service, Hospital—organization & administration.   4. Nursing Staff, Hospital—organization & administration. WY 20.5]
    RA971
    362.17'3068—dc23
                                                                                                2015028125

Printed in the United States of America by Bradford & Bigelow.

CONTENTS

CONTRIBUTORS

Nancy M. Albert, PhD, CCNS, CCRN, NE-BC, FAHA, FCCM, FAAN, Associate Chief Nursing Officer, Office of Nursing Research and Innovation, Nursing Institute, Cleveland Clinic Health System, Cleveland, Ohio; Clinical Nurse Specialist, Kaufman Center for Heart Failure, Cleveland Clinic, Cleveland, Ohio; Adjunct Associate Professor, Case Western Reserve University, Bolton School of Nursing, Cleveland, Ohio; Professor, Aalborg University, Aalborg, Denmark

Cynthia Bautista, PhD, RN, CNRN, SCRN, CCNS, ACNS-BC, FNCS, Neuroscience Clinical Nurse Specialist, Yale–New Haven Hospital, New Haven, Connecticut

Peggy Beat, JD, RN, Attorney and Senior Director, Corporate Compliance, Cleveland Clinic Health System, Cleveland, Ohio

James F. Bena, MS, Lead Biostatistician, Quantitative Health Sciences, Cleveland Clinic Health System, Cleveland, Ohio

Esther I. Bernhofer, PhD, RN-BC, Senior Nurse Researcher, Nursing Institute, Office of Nursing Research and Innovation, Cleveland Clinic Health System, Cleveland, Ohio

Colleen Brooks, BS, Nursing Policy Coordinator, Nursing Research and Evidence-Based Practice Coordinator, Inova Loudoun Hospital, Falls Church, Virginia

Christian Burchill, PhD, RN, CEN, Nurse Researcher, Nursing Institute, Office of Nursing Research and Innovation, Cleveland Clinic Health System, Cleveland, Ohio

Tammy Cupit, PhD, RN-BC, Director, Nursing Research, University of Texas Medical Branch Health System, Galveston, Texas

Roberta Cwynar, MSN, ACNP-BC, Acute Care Nurse Practitioner, Critical Care Transport, Cleveland Clinic Health System, Cleveland, Ohio

Jennifer Fabian, BSN, RN, CCRN, Staff Nurse, Intensive Care Unit, Inova Loudoun Hospital, Leesburg, Virginia

Mary Ann Friesen, PhD, RN, CPHQ, Nursing Research and Evidence-Based Practice Coordinator, Inova Health System, Falls Church, Virginia

Karen Johnson, PhD, RN, Director, Nursing Research, Banner Health, Phoenix, Arizona

Linda J. Lewicki, PhD, RN, CIP, Senior Nurse Researcher, Institutional Review Board, Cleveland Clinic Health System, Cleveland, Ohio

Vicki Lindgren, RN, MSN, CNS, CCRN, CCNS, Clinical Nurse Specialist, Inova Fair Oaks Hospital, Fairfax, Virginia

Mark McClelland, DNP, RN, CPHQ, Nurse Researcher, Nursing Institute, Office of Nursing Research and Innovation, Cleveland Clinic Health System, Cleveland, Ohio

Susan J. McCrudden, BSN, RN, Clinical Nurse, Nursing Institute—Hillcrest Hospital, Cleveland Clinic Health System, Mayfield Heights, Ohio

Laura McNicholl, RN-BC, MS, CNS-BC, Clinical Nurse Specialist, Inova Fair Oaks Hospital, Fairfax, Virginia

Mary Beth Modic, DNP, RN, CDE, Clinical Nurse Specialist, Nursing Education, Office of Education and Professional Practice Development, Cleveland Clinic Health System, Cleveland, Ohio

David Pickham, PhD, RN, Director of Research, Patient Care Services, Stanford Health Care, Stanford, California

Karen L. Rice, DNS, APRN, ACNS-BC, ANP, Director, The Center for Nursing Research, Ochsner Health System, New Orleans, Louisiana

Joel D. Roach, BA, Research Coordinator II, Nursing Institute, Office of Nursing Research and Innovation, Cleveland Clinic Health System, Cleveland, Ohio

Jayne S. Rosenberger, BSN, RN, Clinical Nurse, Nursing Institute—Hillcrest Hospital, Cleveland Clinic Health System, Mayfield Heights, Ohio

Donna M. Ross, MSN, RN, ACNS-BC, CHFN, Clinical Nurse Specialist, Nursing Institute—Lakewood Hospital, Office of Education and Professional Practice Development, Cleveland Clinic Health System, Lakewood, Ohio

Tonya Rutherford-Hemming, EdD, RN, ANP-BC, CHSE, Senior Nurse Researcher, Nursing Institute, Office of Nursing Research and Innovation, Cleveland Clinic Health System, Cleveland, Ohio

Sandra L. Siedlecki, PhD, RN, CNS, Senior Nurse Scientist, Nursing Institute, Office of Nursing Research and Innovation, Cleveland Clinic Health System, Cleveland, Ohio

Jeanne Sorrell, PhD, RN, FAAN, Senior Nurse Scientist (retired), Nursing Institute, Office of Nursing Research and Innovation, Cleveland Clinic Health System, Cleveland, Ohio

Shelley S. Thibeau, PhD, RN-NIC, Senior RN Researcher, The Center for Nursing Research, Ochsner Health System, New Orleans, Louisiana

Connie White-Williams, PhD, RN, FAAN, Director, Center for Nursing Excellence, Assistant Professor, School of Nursing, University of Alabama at Birmingham Hospital, Birmingham, Alabama

PREFACE

This book was developed to appeal to anyone who wants to initiate, nurture, and/or sustain a vibrant hospital or ambulatory care (clinical-based) nursing research program. I have worked at Cleveland Clinic for over 25 years, and I always recall that, throughout that time, we had one nurse researcher (and even two for a short time) whose job it was to lead his or her own program of research and mentor clinical nurses at the main campus. In fact, I used nursing research "services" shortly after being hired as a nurse manager, when I chose to lead my very first clinical research project in 1991. I place quotes around the word "services" because there was no research program or infrastructure—no structures, systems, or processes—and, with a few exceptions, nurses were not encouraged to conduct research. Services consisted of meeting with a doctorate-prepared nurse researcher and getting one-on-one advice. If I had not asked my boss to tell me who could provide assistance, and taken the steps to reach out to the nurse researcher, we would never have connected. I was responsible for leading all communication between us. She mentored me and had great advice, but the relationship was based on what I perceived as my needs—and, as a novice, I really had no clue as to what I needed. I was guessing at every step of the process and trying to read research books (from our hospital library shelves and from my home bookcase of master's program books I had purchased as a student but never really dug into) to get it right. Most clinical nurses did not know that we had this valuable service. When I applied for the job as the director of nursing research, the nursing department had very little research in motion, which explained why nurse researchers were often champions of leadership project work over the years. During the interview, when I asked the chief nursing officer what she was expecting of the director role, she simply stated, "More research; there is no place to go but up!"

Early in the tenure of my role as director of the nursing research department, I began meeting with key supporters of nursing research services: clinical nurse specialists, clinical directors, and nurse managers. There were two lessons learned through these early conversations. First, nurses did not want a nurse researcher to take over their project and become the principal investigator; they wanted to be coached on how to do it right. They considered themselves to be the clinical experts, and they were looking for research expertise. Thus, a nurse researcher did not technically need to be an expert in the nurses' patient population; it was more important to be an expert in nursing research designs, methodologies, and analyses, and in writing research proposals, grants, and publications.

Second, a hospital-based, doctorate-prepared nurse researcher needed to take a different approach from what an academic nurse researcher would take. By this I mean that when hospital nurses are college students completing research for academic degrees, they are self-motivated to continue to completion, as project completion affects graduation status. The nurse researcher is a mentor who offers advice, and it is up to the student to get the work done. That approach may work for determined clinical nurse investigators (after all, it worked for me back in 1991), but it may be very impractical for many hospital-based nurses who need more than a "service." What happens if a library literature search service is not readily available, and even when available, if a nurse has never before completed a literature search or reviewed research abstracts? Hospital-based nurse researchers need to be coaches more often than mentors, and they need to provide research resources *and* assistance to guide nurses toward success. In the process, nurse researchers may become cognitive experts in the fields of study of those with whom they are working, especially when clinical nurses have practical knowledge but not literature-based knowledge in their area of study.

The intent of this book is to provide useful knowledge and practical applications to ease the work of leading or working in a hospital-based nursing research program. This book contains principles that apply to all sizes of hospitals, as well as hospital systems that may be spread out over multiple states or be contained in one area. When I travel, people tell me, "You are from the Cleveland Clinic, and have access to resources that we don't have at our small hospital. Your systems would never work in our hospital." In truth, Cleveland Clinic has large and small hospitals; urban, community, and rural hospitals; hospitals without a single clinical nurse specialist or other nonhourly nurse clinicians who can provide research guidance to clinical nurses. Further, each of our nine hospitals in northeast Ohio and our hospitals in Weston, Florida, and Abu Dhabi serve patient populations that differ in culture, economic circumstances, and community health care resources. We have learned the power of using multiple methods to achieve goals, being open to new ways of producing outcomes, and individualizing our coaching styles based on the needs of the clinical nurse research team, the research project, and available resources.

Like many of you who read this book, when I became the director of nursing research in 2004, I had to confront the fact that there was not much in place in terms of a nursing research program. We had a succession of nurse researchers (as previously stated) who were available to mentor nurses in research, but we did not have a true nursing research program—or, maybe I should say that the nurse researcher *was* the totality of the nursing research program. I had a vision for a nursing research department that was not just about my being available to mentor others. Yes, I wanted to share my passion for nursing research with anyone who was open to listening. Yes, I wanted to mentor and coach nurses who had research questions and a desire to get answers. Yes, I wanted to help clinical nurses, nurse managers, and clinical nurse specialists understand the value of nursing research and the importance of research findings when changing clinical practices. But, more important, I wanted to be a part of something bigger. I wanted to develop a foundation for nursing science within our hospital organization that would facilitate the many processes of research and, ultimately, advance nursing science, locally and globally. Hospital-based nursing research cannot be sustained when it is dependent on one (or more) nurse researcher drivers as its sole resource. It takes a village to make nursing research thrive; it thrives when people, structures, processes, and system resources are available and in alignment with the hospital organization and the vision and mission of nursing leaders.

This book contains 11 chapters. Each is unique in content, and some content may not apply to nursing research programs in all hospitals, depending on the depth and breadth of your program and allowable resources. For example, your hospital may use a shared governance research council as the primary structure to lead nursing research initiatives, or your hospital may not have its own institutional review board. Even when content does not seem to match your structure and available resources, content within a particular chapter will give you new ideas and strategies that can benefit your program. Chapter authors are all experts in their respective fields. In most chapters, they combine practical clinical knowledge with relevant literature, and in many chapters, tables and figures are provided as a visual guide to enhance the words. Within the nursing research program at Cleveland Clinic, we developed many resources to assist nurse researchers and nurse investigators. To share content with you in the most practical way, we displayed the first page of multipage tables and figures. In this way, as readers, you are guided by viewing the formatting and words. To obtain full tables and figures, readers are encouraged to go to www.onadeo.com, a marketplace devoted to bringing world-class solutions to colleagues.

Nancy M. Albert

ACKNOWLEDGMENTS

This book was conceived years ago when one of my colleagues, Sandra Siedlecki, and I were discussing the people we have met along our nursing research journeys and their desires for support in developing or sustaining a nursing research program. We came to realize that many nurses were asking similar questions. We felt we could support and encourage those who were working toward specific milestones and we wanted to share our accomplishments with others, in hopes that their programs could reach a high level of success. Our conversations spurred us both to raise again the possibility of writing a book, and our fuel for making it happen was the many phone and in-person consultations we have had with master's- or doctorate-prepared nurse researchers who made statements such as, "I wish I had this book right now!" I thank all of the nurses I have consulted with over the years, as your search for answers and comments about your nursing research services became the basis for content of the chapters of this book.

This book was a team effort by my nursing research colleagues at the Cleveland Clinic, including nurses, a research coordinator, a biostatistician, and a research compliance officer. Their devotion to their professions and willingness to take time to write their chapters was very much appreciated. Special thanks to Jeanne Sorrell, who worked with me to lay out the content themes for each chapter, and to all chapter writers for creating content not found in other nursing research books. Also, thanks to authors for meeting deadlines and being open to adding and subtracting content as the book took shape. In total there are 28 contributors to this book, many of whom provide content for the "Voices of Nurse Researchers" segments that are interwoven within chapters. These short segments provide useful knowledge and recommendations from hospital-based nurses throughout the country. Their voices provide pragmatic advice and examples of considerations that led to their nursing research successes. I am tremendously thankful that they took time to share their stories, many of which augment the words of chapter writers.

I thank K. Kelly Hancock, our executive chief nursing officer and chief nursing officer of the main campus, for her many contributions to the success of our nursing research program. Early after I shared my plans to develop a nursing research program that was more than just a communication service (in 2004), Kelly, who at the time was a clinical director, communicated the need to conduct nursing research to her clinical department managers and leaders. Kelly was one of many clinical directors, yet it was her early support of nursing research and our team's mission that led to an influx of research projects led by clinical nurses within her department. Those early research projects taught my team a lot about the needs of clinicians when juggling clinical work and nursing research, and helped us to establish resources to meet clinician needs. More importantly, nonmaster's-degree clinical nurses became the faces of rigorous nursing research projects. Today, Kelly is an inspirational leader for nurses and nursing at Cleveland Clinic. Her unwavering leadership and support of generating and using new knowledge gained through nursing research to advance nursing and ensure we are truly providing best practices permeate our mission, strategic plans, and allocation of resources.

Finally, and most important, I wish to recognize my husband, Gerard, my daughters, Samantha, Alyssa, and Stephanie, and my future son-in-law, Bill, for their patience and emotional support as I toiled through the writing and chapter reviews of this book. Blending my passion for getting this book completed with my desire and need for family time did not always balance out, but my family brought me back to reality with regular visits into my home office, and challenges to break for dinners, exercise, and shared activities. I love you all; you are simply wonderful!

Mark McClelland
Nancy M. Albert

1

CREATING A VISION FOR NURSING RESEARCH BY UNDERSTANDING BENEFITS

In this opening chapter, we begin by answering the question: What are the benefits of a nursing research program? We describe how nursing research provides new evidence for nursing practice that improves clinical outcomes, changes the culture of the organization, creates new leadership roles for nurses, offers opportunities for interdisciplinary collaboration, enhances patient safety, improves nurse and patient satisfaction, and leads to positive branding of the hospital and the nursing department. As the health care industry transitions from a volume-based to a value-based payment system, it is imperative that nursing leadership recognizes the benefits of initiating, growing, and sustaining a nursing research program. Nursing leadership can create (or support) a vision for nursing research based on the benefits that are central to the hospital's strategic mission and goals.

BENEFITS OF NURSING RESEARCH

Nursing Research Provides New Evidence for Nursing Practice

Nurses are ideally positioned to design, develop, and conduct research on patient and caregiver interventions and new protocols, pathways, tools, and processes, and then, to implement important evidence-based interventions in clinical settings. In addition to individual nursing research reports published in peer-reviewed journals, there are many global examples in the literature of how nursing research can create new ideas that can improve nursing science, transform nursing practice, and be translated into policy. Four examples that can be used to energize nurses to the power of nursing research are provided. First, the National Institute of Nursing Research published a report of 10 landmark nursing research studies that changed practice over time (National Institute of Nursing Research, 2006). Second, members of the National Nursing Research Roundtable (Grady & Gullatte, 2014) published a report of the science of caregiving that included multiple nursing research themes of importance in moving the science forward, such as dementia, sleep disturbance, caregiving across the life span (family-oriented interventions), nurse-facilitated conversation, and providing health information. Third, in one issue of a Robert Wood Johnson Foundation publication, 11 research reports on the following themes were discussed in relation to nursing research: quality of care, patient safety, reliable care, cost and value of nursing time in improving clinical outcomes, changing the environment of care, enhancing the pool of qualified clinical nurses, balancing nurse staffing costs and adverse outcomes, supportive workforce, and patient-centered care (Grace, 2006). Finally, the Interdisciplinary Nursing Quality Research Initiative (INQRI) of the Robert Wood Johnson Foundation was developed to promote more research that shows the impact of nursing. Themes of importance to INQRI are those that advance understanding of the nursing process, workforce, and environment; the effects of innovation on quality of patient care; hospital-based (acute care) structural, organizational, and environmental factors that affect quality of nursing care delivery; how quality of nursing care is measured accurately in ways that are useful and feasible; and methods that specifically improve nursing and patient outcomes based on changes in the nursing workplace or workforce (www.inqri.org). In a 2012 report from the Robert Wood Johnson Foundation, examples of research themes that could directly affect nursing practices were the effect of patient activation on pain self-management, use of information technology to resolve medication discrepancies in home care, medical–surgical nurse workload and characteristics on patient outcomes, use of a fall prevention bundle to decrease hospital falls, and an interdisciplinary nurse-led plan to decrease delirium in critically ill adults (Naylor, Pauly, & Melichar, 2012). Thus, hospital-based nursing research has the power to transform nursing care and lead to patient, nurse, and hospital benefits. A well-developed and executed nursing research program will create an infrastructure that guides nurses toward improving their practice.

All too often hospital care that is delivered should not be, and care that is not delivered, should be. Your reading of this book is evidence that nurses are making progress in their quest to provide better care to individuals, improve the health of populations, and lower the costs of care using evidence-based practices (EBP) and research. The Institute of Medicine (IOM, 2011) set a goal that by 2020, 90% of all health care decisions should be guided by evidence. Melnyk, Fineout-Overholt, Gallagher-Ford, and Kaplan (2012) reported that between the years 2005 and 2013 clinical nurses became ready to adopt EBP, yet authors also pointed out that well-known barriers to basing practice on

TABLE 1.1 Barriers and Facilitators to Using Evidence-Based Practices in Nursing and
Conducting Nursing Research

BARRIERS	FACILITATORS
• Time limitations/heavy workloads/staffing issues • Organizational culture relies on tradition and maintaining outdated work/practices • Inadequate EBP education and skill training • Have not taken a research course; lack of knowledge of and confidence in using research • Lack of access to databases • Lack of support by managers and leaders • Resistance from nursing and medical colleagues • Lack of understanding of how to critically appraise evidence • Intimidated by research • Nursing research is not a priority • Lack of an institutional research infrastructure • Do not understand or value research • Lack of relevance to nursing practice • Lack of interest	• Education/research training • Access to information clearinghouse for evidence-based information • Dedicated time • Organizational support/awareness • Manager support • Mentors available on unit; nursing research mentors • Written EBP standards of practice • Making research relevant • Peer and physician support • Money to support EBP and research initiatives • Increased awareness of the importance of EBP • Tangible research resources • Research is part of the job • Nursing research council

EBP, evidence-based practice.

evidence and conducting nursing research remained consistent and strong after 20 years of discussion. Table 1.1 provides barriers to and facilitators of using EBP and conducting nursing research that were identified by clinical nurses and nurse leaders (Kelly, Turner, Speroni, McLaughlin, & Guzzetta, 2013; Melnyk et al., 2012; Packerton et al., 2009; Pravikoff, Tanner, & Pierce, 2005; Smirnoff, Ramirez, Kooplimae, Gibney, & McEvoy, 2007; Yoder et al., 2014). To ensure that patient outcomes and administrative decisions that affect nursing practices are based on the highest level of research evidence available and to increase the conduct and consumption of nursing research by clinical nurses, there is a need for education, information, and support. A nursing research program will provide the necessary education, information, and support needed to enhance facilitators and minimize barriers to searching, appraising, and using research literature, translating research results into clinical practice, and conducting new nursing research that leads to implementation of EBP.

Complexity of nursing care has increased over time due to medical discoveries, improved technological capacity and communication methods, regulatory expectations, and the speed with which changes occur. So, too, patient complexity has increased as patients live longer, are more likely to have multiple comorbidities, and bear an increasing share of the costs of care. Nursing practice must evolve to keep pace with the changing landscape of hospital care and the national push for value-based care (high-quality care and outcomes at lower cost), and autonomous, accountable nursing practice. A strong scientific foundation, combined with a professional practice model that is founded on EBP and research will help nurses meet and exceed stakeholder goals and consumer expectations (River, Cohen, & Counsell, 2006).

As with most social change, hospital-based clinical nurses and nursing leaders must be *willing* and *able* to take the leap toward an EBP infrastructure. The American Nurse Credentialing Center Magnet® program designation has focused on clinical nurses' participation in nursing research and use of EBP. Magnet-designated hospitals were more likely to have higher patient safety and quality of care in the United States (Witkoski Stimpfel, Rosen, & McHugh, 2014) and internationally (Cheung, Aiken, Clarke, & Sloane, 2008), providing evidence that attention to professional practice through EBP and nursing research has important implications.

Nursing Research Changes the Culture of an Organization

Important clues for detecting an organization's predominant culture are its visible structures and processes (artifacts). The organizational structures and processes put in place by top leadership are a reflection of current priorities and serve as constant communication of what they want their employees to pay attention to (Schein, 2012). For instance, if a hospital states that it values patient and family input, one would expect to see multiple avenues throughout the hospital that facilitate consumer feedback. Many hospitals purport to support interdisciplinary care, but historically, nurses' experiences in interdisciplinary patient rounds were suboptimal. Scott and Pollock (2008) reported that during patient rounds, nurses would report objective findings but not necessarily contribute to the development of the patient care plan. "You know, keep your head down. Do what you're told," commented one nurse about her role in rounds (p. 302). A hospital-based nursing research program creates a driver to counterbalance medical authority and hierarchical leadership, a cultural dynamic still prevalent in too many hospitals. By committing funding and resources to research, the chief nursing officer (CNO) shows concern for the evidence base of the many policies and procedures governing nursing, which then serves as an example to staff that they too should be concerned about the evidence base of their units' standards of care. This alignment sets the tone for an evidence-based culture.

When nurses are incentivized to work in an evidence-based culture, translation and dissemination of EBP and nursing research thrives. The best chance of success in nursing research is a culture supported from the top down but driven by a bottom-up approach (The Advisory Board Company, 2003). In a bottom-up approach, clinical nurses are knowledgeable about EBP and have support to seek out best practice evidence, question nursing practices and policies for strength and quality of evidence, consider new ways of carrying out nursing practice, develop questions amenable to research, and expect to methodically derive answers to these questions through research. Although a research study, with its rigor and design considerations, is usually a deliberate, slow-paced activity affecting few staff, and the impact on culture change is commensurately slow, an immediate and powerful cultural driver of a research program is that the status, use, and demand for actionable research-based evidence is greatly elevated.

An executive nurse champion, in-hospital research leadership, and a program of EBP/research awareness among clinical nurses create and sustain internal expertise that will initiate a cultural change away from "tradition" and "we have always done it this way" modes of thinking. When the professional practice model visibly empowers nurses to seek knowledge and deliver validated care that promotes high quality outcomes, a culture that supports research will become more prevalent. Ultimately, nursing will have a larger stake in contributing to an evidence-based culture that resonates throughout the hospital. The nursing research program becomes a very visible and accountable stakeholder that advocates for EBP—even across disciplines.

VOICE OF A NURSE RESEARCHER

David Pickham, PhD, RN
Director of Research, Patient Care Services, Stanford Health Care,
Stanford, California

In building a program of research, many resources are needed. Many of these are negotiable: time, space, budget, and so on. What is not negotiable, and is critical to developing a successful program of research, is the support of nursing leadership and specifically the support of the CNO.

In any organization, strategic priorities drive the provision of resources. At Stanford, and surely throughout the United States, our mission is to continually increase the "value" we provide to our patients. Therefore, we see anything that doesn't add value to patients as being wasteful. For a program of research to be successful within an organization, I believe it is imperative to first align the research program with both the nursing and the organization's strategic plans. If this is successfully completed, research will be seen as adding value to the clinical care environment. The CNO can then advocate for and provide the necessary programmatic support for the research program.

Nursing Research Creates New Leadership Roles for Nurses

Prior to the global health care practice movement, whereby clinical decisions are based on evidence, hospital nursing services made nursing practice decisions using tradition, physician authority, and trial and error. Increasingly, governmental agencies, regulatory bodies, insurance companies, and national specialty organizations are pushing hospitals to identify, evaluate, and implement EBP. Nurses gaining skills in EBP and research methods will emerge as informal leaders in pursuit of clinical excellence within their work groups. As nurses gain expert status and become EBP gurus, they will be recognized as "go-to" people about EBP, and may find themselves being drawn into policy and procedure committees, nursing research teams, patient education task forces, quality improvement workgroups, and other initiatives that enhance quality outcomes. Activities associated with EBP expertise may be used as evidence for clinical ladder advancement or in annual performance reviews. More important, informal leaders who maintain their expertise status by accessing up-to-date best practices and research evidence will essentially become supportive infrastructure sponsors of EBP. As sponsors of EBP, informal leaders can comfortably facilitate decision making and improved clinical care within daily huddles with colleagues and in local interdisciplinary team rounds.

As nursing research within the hospital grows and formal EBP governance structures expand (see Chapter 4), nurses will have new opportunities to advance in leadership roles, including formal roles as dashboard managers, outcome managers, or quality analysts, or in multiple roles in a formal research program. Stevens (2013) identified the emerging fields of translational and improvement science, implementation research, and health delivery systems science as natural offshoots of implementing a formal nursing research program. As publications of research and quality outcomes become visible externally, nurses who are clinical scholars, are EBP experts, and lead clinical research may be called upon to give expert advice regionally or nationally. All these endeavors provide opportunities for nurses to develop important, clinically based leadership roles.

Nursing Research Offers Opportunities for Interdisciplinary Collaboration

One of the five core competencies for health care providers proscribed by the IOM (Greiner & Knebel, 2003) is the ability to work in interdisciplinary teams. EBP is the future currency of health care, and discovering, describing, debating, and delivering evidence will be the primary purpose of interdisciplinary hospital teams. Health care, particularly within hospitals, has been traditionally organized around multidisciplinary teams; each discipline focusing on its part of the patient, always working sequentially or in parallel with other disciplines. Authority and leadership were typically vested in physicians, and the focus was on communication, not collaboration, leading to multiple plans of care. In contrast, interdisciplinary teams work to meet multiple patient needs and priorities by integrating care plans from all disciplines into a single plan of care. Team members accept leadership from the most knowledgeable team member and learn to trust each other to achieve patient goals (Heinemann & Zeiss, 2002).

The mainstay of interdisciplinary collaboration is patient rounds. In a review of literature, patient rounds were associated with positive patient outcomes (Epstein, 2014) and were valued by many nurses and some physicians (Gonzalo, Kuperman, Lehman, & Haidet, 2014). A prerequisite to interdisciplinary collaboration is nurses' ability to effectively speak and understand the language of research. Research literacy is the ability to locate, understand, and appraise evidence for application in practice (Nolan & Behi, 1996). An organized, proactive nursing research program will help clinical nurses develop the research literacy needed to contribute intellectually and assertively during interdisciplinary patient care planning rounds.

Interdisciplinary research has gained popularity since funders and scientific organizations began discussing enhancing disciplinary integration to promote scientific advances. In nursing, interdisciplinarity can become very important, since medical advances require nursing input for successful implementation and nursing advances generally require collaboration during translation. The Affordable Care Act of 2010 created and generously funded the Patient-Centered Outcomes Research Institute (PCORI; Frank Basch, & Selby, 2014), a nonprofit, nongovernmental organization authorized by the U.S. Congress. PCORI's mission is to prioritize and fund clinical comparative effectiveness research that will lead to improved patient outcomes. Due to nursing's pivotal role and proximity to patients, PCORI is committed to increasing nurses' contribution to interdisciplinary collaboration in research (www.pcori .org/events/2014/pcori-practice-highlighting-opportunities-nurses). Further, the Agency for Healthcare Research and Quality (AHRQ), one of the largest governmental funders of research, made a call for interdisciplinary teams, including consumers, to identify, measure, and answer important research questions (Stevens, 2013). Interdisciplinary research is still in its infancy; the dynamics of disciplinary integration science require more knowledge (Adams & Light, 2014). In a Cochrane review of interventions intended to increase interdisciplinary collaboration, researchers found only a few studies that addressed the topic (Zwarenstein, Goldman, & Reeves, 2009). Due to multiple study limitations, Cochrane review authors labeled the evidence as promising rather than proven and called for more research. Nurses acting as patient advocates have an obligation to provide evidence-based interventions that promote optimization of interdisciplinary care.

Nursing Research Improves Nurse and Patient Satisfaction

The IOM supports protecting the public from harm. Use of highest strength EBP and nursing research findings may have benefits in changing nurses' work environment and the delivery of health care, which may ultimately improve patient safety and outcomes (MacDavitt, Cieplinski, & Walker, 2011) and promote patient satisfaction. Moreover, when nurses have a voice in decision making, they create influence and control over their practice, and enhance job satisfaction. Having a voice in nursing research creates an environment that fosters autonomy and interdisciplinary collaboration that may also enhance nurse satisfaction (Grace, 2006; MacDavitt et al., 2011; Rivers, Cohen, & Counsell, 2006).

Nursing research involves data, and data are highly prevalent in many formats in today's world of informatics, including data from internet sites, hospital databases, electronic medical records, billing systems, national guidelines, and Cochrane reviews. Data, when converted into information through analysis and interpretation, are used to safeguard patients, align nursing practices with the realities of patient care, develop new ideas and innovations, make decisions, and challenge current practices, to name a few (Douglas, 2014). When research is an integral component of nursing departments, nurses will understand how to access, validate, analyze, interpret, and use data to develop solutions, promote best practices, and improve administrative functions, all of which could enhance nurse and patient satisfaction.

Nursing Research Promotes Branding for the Hospital and Nursing Department

In the literature outlining the benefits of nursing research, branding of the hospital and, more specifically, the nursing department is not discussed. However, consider this scenario: A nurse at your hospital conducts a research study on a topic of high interest to nursing practice. The research resulted in practice changes in the hospital and was published in a peer-reviewed journal. You wisely had your marketing department develop a story about study findings for a hospital publication that is shared with community health care leaders. Within months of the publication, a few things begin to happen: (a) nurse administrators call the hospital to learn more about the research intervention and/or practice change; (b) nurses from other hospitals make requests to spend time at your hospital (to see evidence of the intervention/practice change and factors that affected implementation); (c) your nurse authors are invited to speak at national and regional meetings on the theme, specific research methods, and results; (d) nurse authors are asked for input on implications and next steps related to the research theme (clinical scholar) and to participate as a consultant on related projects in start-ups at other hospitals; and (e) nurses are asked to participate as members of national committees or task forces, which may result in papers and organization policies on research theme content, or implications may be included in scientific statements or guidelines. All of the above brand your hospital, nursing department, and research nurses as thematic or service line experts. Moreover, nonhospital nurses may have more positive perceptions of nursing departments in branded hospitals. Positive differentiation could ease nurse recruitment efforts, especially if the nursing department also has national awards, Magnet designation status, highly rated physicians, cutting-edge technology, and community and national consumer awareness. Nurse retention directly increases a hospital's "intellectual property" of best nursing practices that could promote improved patient outcomes. Further, costs of recruitment and orientation will be reduced.

VOICE OF A NURSE RESEARCHER

David Pickham, PhD, RN
Director of Research, Patient Care Services, Stanford Health Care, Stanford, California

As our nursing research program continues to grow, the perception of nursing research across the campus is also changing. What I found at the beginning is that often people do not quite understand what nursing research is—and it is not their fault. We have spent a lot of time as a profession trying to define our body of knowledge, often without consensus. We have complicated education structures (multiple credentials at the bachelor's, master's, and doctorate levels) and professional clinical roles. It is no wonder others find it hard to understand what nursing research is. Often, the perception is simply that nurses do not really do research.

But as we continue to build nursing research, important changes are occurring. Outsiders to nursing are beginning to understand what research within nursing is and the role research has in the profession. With staff undertaking research and speaking with colleagues, research is increasingly being seen as something that is accessible, relevant, and valuable to clinical practice. A successful nursing research program is one of the best advertisements the profession can have within an organization.

REFERENCES

Adams, J., & Light, R. (2014). Mapping interdisciplinary fields: Efficiencies, gaps and redundancies in HIV/AIDS research. *PLoS One, 9*(12), e115092.

The Advisory Board Company. (2003). Toward evidence-based nursing: Reforming culture, enhancing practice. Washington, DC: Author.

Cheung, R. B., Clarke, L. H., Aiken, S. P., & Sloane, D. M. (2008). Nursing care and patient outcomes: International evidence. *Enfermería Clínica, 18*(1), 5–40.

Douglas, K. (2014). How data is changing our world. *Nurse Leader, 12*(5), 37–39, 67.

Epstein, N. E. (2014). Multidisciplinary in-hospital teams improve patient outcomes: A review. *Surgical Neurology International. 5*(Supplement 7), S295–S303.

Frank, L., Basch, E., & Selby, J. V. (2014). The PCORI perspective on patient-centered outcomes research. *Journal of the American Medical Association, 312*(15), 1513–1514.

Gonzalo, J. D., Kuperman, E., Lehman, E., & Haidet, P. (2014). Bedside interprofessional rounds: Perceptions of benefits and barriers by internal medicine nursing staff, attending physicians, and housestaff physicians. *Journal of Hospital Medicine, 9*(10), 646–651.

Grace, J. A. (2006). *New research that illuminates policy issues: Balancing nursing costs and quality of care for patients. Charting nursing's future.* Robert Wood Johnson Foundation: http://www.rwjf.org/en/research-publications/find-rwjf-research/2009/01/charting-nursings-future-archives/new-research-that-illuminates-policy-issues.html

Grady, P. A., & Gullatte, M. (2014). The 2014 national nursing research roundtable: The science of caregiving. *Nursing Outlook, 62*(5), 362–365.

Greiner, A. C., & Knebel, E. (Eds.). (2003). *Health professions education: A bridge to quality.* Institute of Medicine (IOM). Washington, DC: National Academies Press.

Heinemann, G. D., & Zeiss, A. M. (Eds.). (2002). *Team performance in health care: Assessment and development.* New York, NY: Kluwer Academic/Plenum Publishers.

Institute of Medicine (IOM). (2011). *Engineering a Learning Healthcare System: A Look at the Future: Workshop Summary.* Washington, DC: The National Academies Press.

Kelly, K. P., Turner, A., Gabel Speroni, K., McLaughlin, M. K., & Guzzetta, C. E. (2013). National survey of hospital nursing research, part 2: Facilitators and hindrances. *Journal of Nursing Administration, 43*(1), 18–23.

Melnyk, B. M., Fineout-Overholt, E., Gallagher-Ford, L., & Kaplan, L. (2012). The state of evidence-based practice in U.S. nurses: Critical implications for nurse leaders and educators. *Journal of Nursing Administration, 42*(9), 410–417.

National Institute of Nursing Research. (2006). Changing practice, changing lives: 10 landmark nursing studies. *U.S. Department of Health and Human Services.* (Bethesda MD): NIH Publication number 06–6094. http://www.ninr.nih.gov/sites/www.ninr.nih.gov/files/10-landmark-nursing-research-studies.pdf

Naylor, M. D., Pauly, M. V., & Melichar, L. (2012). *Interdisciplinary Research that Demonstrates the Role of Nurses in Improving the Quality of Care.* Robert Wood Johnson Foundation. Retrieved from http://www.rwjf.org/en/library/research/ 2012/05/interdisciplinary-research-that-demonstrates-the-role-of--nurses.html

Nolan, M., & Behi, R. (1996). From methodology to method: The building blocks of research literacy. *British Journal of Nursing, 5,* 54–57.

Packerton, P. H., Needleman, J., Pearson, M. L., Upenieks, V. V., Soban, L. M., & Yee, T. (2009). Lessons from nursing leaders on implementing TCAB. *American Journal of Nursing, 109*(11, Supplement), 71–76.

Patient Centered Outcomes Research Institute. (2014). *PCORI in Practice: Highlighting Opportunities for Nurses.* Webinar. http://www.pcori.org/events/2014/pcori-practice-highlighting-opportunities-nurses

Pravikoff, D. S., Tanner, A. B., & Pierce, S. T. (2005). Readiness of U.S. nurses for evidence-based practice. *American Journal of Nursing, 105*(9), 40–51.

Rivers, R., Cohen, L., & Counsell, C. (2006). Science: Critical to patient care. *Nurse Leader, 4*(3), 40–44.

Schein, E. H. (2012). *Organizational Culture and Leadership* (4th ed.). San Francisco, CA: Jossey-Bass.

Scott, S. D., & Pollock, C. (2008). The role of nursing unit culture in shaping research utilization behaviors. *Research in Nursing & Health, 31,* 298–309.

Smirnoff, M., Ramirez, M., Kooplimae, L., Gibney, M., & McEvoy, M. D. (2007). Nurses' attitudes toward nursing research at a metropolitan medical center. *Applied Nursing Research, 20*(1), 24–31.

Stevens, K. (2013). The impact of evidence-based practice in nursing and the next big ideas. *OJIN: The Online Journal of Issues in Nursing, 18*(2). Manuscript 4.

Witkoski Stimpfel, A., Rosen, J. E., & McHugh, M. (2014). Understanding the role of the professional practice environment on quality of care in Magnet® and non-Magnet hospitals. *Journal of Nursing Administration, 44*(1), 10–16.

Yoder, L. H., Kirkley, D., McFall, D. C., Kirksey, K. M., StalBaum, A. L., & Sellers, D. (2014). Staff nurses' use of research to facilitate evidence-based practice. *American Journal of Nursing, 114*(9), 26–37.

Zwarenstein, M., Goldman, J., & Reeves, S. (2009). Interprofessional collaboration: Effects of practice-based interventions on professional practice and healthcare outcomes. *Cochrane Database of Systematic Reviews, 2009* (3). doi: 10.1002/14651858 .CD000072.pub2

Nancy M. Albert

2

PLANNING AND IMPLEMENTING A CLINICAL RESEARCH PROGRAM INFRASTRUCTURE

This chapter focuses specifically on nursing research program vertical infrastructure. Vertical infrastructure refers to the pillars of the program: the foundation that provides the support to build other services. Three essential components are used to develop a solid nursing research program foundation that advances the scientific foundation of nursing practice and promotes integration of evidence-based practices. The three components are nurse researchers who coach or mentor clinical nurses in nursing research, intranet website resources, and a research departmental database. Any hospital, regardless of size or affiliation, can have a flourishing, sustainable nursing research program. It is our hope that the information in this chapter will get you excited about building and sustaining a nursing research program at your hospital. If you already have a nursing research program, the information presented will give you new ideas about how you can nurture your program toward continued success and sustainability and even new growth.

It is important to set a strong vertical structure or foundation early on, so that costs of business, personnel needs, and increased capacity are known and manageable over time. A nursing research program may start small and involve a single nurse who is designated to make nursing research happen. Alternately, nursing leadership may designate a nurse researcher leader to develop a business plan for a program with expectations that it grows over time. Thus, the foundational elements discussed herein can apply to both a large or small nursing research program.

An essential element of setting the foundation and planning, growing, and nurturing a nursing research program is to demonstrate how the program aligns with the strategic plan (vision, mission, and goals) of nursing. Further, learning the vision, mission, and goals of the hospital will help the nursing research program align from the top on down. Creating a business plan that is in alignment with leadership strategic goals will create synergies of purpose and increase the meaningfulness and importance of the research program. Table 2.1 provides nursing leadership strategic themes that can be enhanced by an active, vibrant research program.

The three foundational elements of strong nursing research programs— personnel, intranet resources, and a nursing research department database, as seen in Figure 2.1—are interconnected and should be available to the entire nursing department, including non-nurse providers and administrators, because important research questions can come from anyone on the team.

TABLE 2.1 Synergy Between Nursing Leadership Strategic Goals and a Nursing Research Program

LEADERSHIP STRATEGIC GOALS	NURSING RESEARCH PROGRAM RELEVANCE
Clinical: Excellent Outcomes	• Creates new knowledge that advances clinical care and global health • Provides high level of strength and quality of evidence that supports clinical initiatives • Answers questions that are currently based on expert/consensus opinion
Clinical: Patient Safety	• Creates new knowledge about how to increase or maintain quality and patient safety • Provides outcome data that reinforce the value of nursing practices and provides evidence for changes in practice, capital and operating purchases, and novel interventions to improve hospital and postdischarge safety • Longitudinal data analysis of important outcomes provides ongoing evidence of expectations
Clinical: Patient/ Family Engagement/ Activation	• Leads to new/advanced strategies that promote better health, improved quality of life and end-of-life, facilitate patient preferences, and lead to improved patient satisfaction • Promotes development and use of clinically relevant tools that measure patient-centered outcomes

Caregiver: Competent Workforce	• Outcomes can impact decisions related to hospital and unit orientation and continuing education in various areas—informatics, nursing practice, charge nurse, middle management, and leadership—and can be related to:
	  ▪ Time to outcomes
	  ▪ Consistency in meeting expectations

Employee Engagement and Care Provider Retention	• Professionalism through research may meet personal/professional goals that increase job satisfaction and retention
	• Promotes new knowledge from:
	  ▪ Review of literature
	  ▪ Research analysis
	  ▪ Research implications
	• Promotes higher education (formally or informally), and shared governance decision making

Workplace Safety/ Quality	• Personal work safety, workplace violence, workplace bullying, and other related safety/quality themes are sensitive topics, amenable to both qualitative and quantitative research

(continued)

TABLE 2.1 Synergy Between Nursing Leadership Strategic Goals and a Nursing
Research Program (*continued*)

LEADERSHIP STRATEGIC GOALS	NURSING RESEARCH PROGRAM RELEVANCE
Value-Based Purchasing	• Rigorous quality and cost of care data can expose disparities and gaps in care and outcomes • Rehospitalization, postdischarge mortality, quality of life, and other clinical outcomes of hospitalization provide strong evidence of the value of patient management pathways and care plans • Research results can promote new revenue streams, cost efficiencies, and innovation
Innovation	• Research and innovation are closely linked; research can lead to innovation and innovative ideas, and inventions generally require research-based outcomes before ready for generalizable use

Academic Partnerships	• Collaborative research enhances:
	   ▪ Resources
	   ▪ Innovation
	• Collaborative research leads to:
	   ▪ Transformational experiences and change
	   ▪ Knowledge generation

Interdisciplinary Collaboration	• When initiated or advanced through research, creates a healthy work environment, fosters lifelong learning about other disciplines, promotes crucial conversations that advance practice and solve problems (especially related to translating new knowledge into practice)

Professional Practice	• Refined through research
	• Research promotes:
	   ▪ EBP knowledge
	   ▪ Professional /scholarly reform

EBP, evidence-based practice.

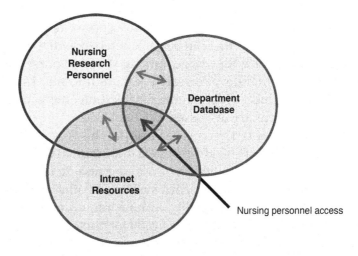

FIGURE 2.1 Foundational elements to initiating, growing, and sustaining nursing research programs.

The three elements of Figure 2.1 are "foundational," based on our experiences in nursing research program development and growth at the Cleveland Clinic Health System in Cleveland, Ohio.

When the department was reorganized to be independent of other departments in May 2004, Cleveland Clinic's main campus was part of a network of hospitals but functioned independently of the health system. The Cleveland Clinic was not involved academically in partnership with a university-based nursing program; we did not have academic nurses steeped in nursing science readily available to us. In 2004, there were no foundational pieces in place, with the exception of one doctorate-prepared nurse researcher. The nurse researcher had been mentoring nurses in research for many years, when requests came through. However, outcomes were limited as there was only one funded nursing research study in progress (co-led by her and a clinical nurse specialist) and a few in start-up discussions when the department was born. Despite researcher availability as a mentor, approximately 3,500 clinical nursing personnel at the main campus, availability of master's-prepared clinical nurse specialists, global nurse leadership support of nursing research, and a high prevalence of physician-led clinical research, very little nursing research was in progress or previously completed. Table 2.2 provides the end-of-year nursing research process and outcomes growth for the first seven years after initiating the three foundational elements at the Cleveland Clinic main campus. Each foundational element is defined briefly.

Personnel: These are researchers who coach and mentor nursing personnel involved in research processes. For larger hospitals that have multiple research projects in process at one time, personnel include other gatekeepers needed to maintain program services and ensure quality in conducting, disseminating, and translating research and in protecting human subjects.

Intranet Resources: These include the internal hospital organization's online templates, checklists, forms, handouts, intranet site links, and communication that nursing personnel can easily access. As the sophistication of the research program grows, so too will the scope of resources. Of note, there are many other resources that can be considered essential, especially to large hospital organizations with a large nursing staff and nurse leadership who have expectations of high-level research (e.g., multicenter randomized controlled trials) that produce widely generalizable outcome evidence. Other nursing research resources are discussed in Chapter 3.

Nursing Research Department Database: This is an electronic system of input and storage of direct and indirect data important to the development, conduct, translation, and dissemination of nursing research. This definition does not refer to electronic medical record systems or other electronic databases supported by the hospital for quality, administration, accounting, or statistical purposes. Rather, it is a database specifically for nurse researchers, research program leaders, and nursing leadership, as it provides evidence of current and previously completed research "knowledge work." Other database resources that help to build a nursing research program are discussed in Chapter 3.

TABLE 2.2 End-of-Year Nursing Research Process and Outcomes Growth at the Main Campus of Cleveland Clinic; First Seven Years

METRICS	YEAR						
	2004	2005	2006	2007	2008	2009	2010
Research Process Growth							
IRB approved[a]	10	25	47	36	27	49	57
In Process[b]	14	67	34	20	17	20	25
Research Outcomes Growth, Frequencies							
Active Research[c]	24	92	81	56	44	69	82
Completed Research	1	7	14	16	19	10	10
Research Presentations[d]	0	2	2	10	14	14	11
Research Publications; First Author/ Total Author Listing[e]	0/0	0/1	1/2	4/13	6/16	12/25	12/20
Nurse Researcher FTEs	1.2	4.0	4.0	3.5	3.0	1.5	3.0

[a]Includes IRB approved projects, projects using data in the public domain, and projects deemed by the IRB to be quality, but were considered quality research studies.

[b]Projects in startup (research question developed and proposal in development). Prior to the end of 2006, we eliminated "in process" projects from the active file of the research department database that were initiated but never moved forward to IRB approval.

[c]Includes IRB approved and in-process nurse-led research projects.

[d]At regional, national, or international meetings.

[e]Reflects nurse authored research papers in peer-reviewed journals.

FTE, full time equivalent; IRB, institutional review board.

The three foundational elements of nurse researcher personnel, intranet resources, and a departmental research database are discussed in the following sections in detail, and include element descriptions and features that can be replicated by other hospital organizations. Insights from staff input during interviews and lessons learned from our experiences over time are included.

NURSE RESEARCHER PERSONNEL

A successful nursing research program is contingent on having the right nurse researcher personnel who can move research from project inception to dissemination in peer-reviewed literature and translation into practice.

There are no research-based reports available on right-sizing of nursing research personnel or the right qualities of personnel. The following characteristics and capabilities of personnel are based on our experiences over time and the published experiences of hospital-based nursing research program directors.

First, nursing researcher productivity (quantity and quality of nurse-led research and dissemination) is higher when people selected are those with a history of and a passion for developing, leading, managing, and disseminating nursing research as a principal investigator (PI), beyond research that was part of a college graduate program that led to an academic degree. Passion may be exhibited as a history of submitting and receiving grants, conducting research when grant dollars are not available, working with multiple types of analyses, writing papers on personal time (rather than work time) to move dissemination forward and prevent stagnation of new knowledge, receiving and successfully responding to journal peer-reviewer feedback, and looking for and participating in valuable experiences that facilitate strong research processes and minimize unnecessary work. Nurse researchers with passion are internally driven and self-motivated to produce high quality research and demonstrate serving-leader characteristics when coaching and mentoring nurses in research. In oral conversations, passionate nurse researchers light up when asked to discuss nursing research, verbalize their thoughts with depth and breadth of knowledge, and show exuberance or animation when discussing mentorship of others.

Often, nurse researchers work as a solo position, especially in small hospitals. Nurse researchers with a passion for nursing research (in general) display eagerness in working on research concepts and in patient populations in which they do not have expertise, merely because the research question and hypothesis are intriguing, and they enjoy the research process. Since colleagues are not readily available for consultation, it is imperative that nurse researchers seek out requisite knowledge needed to advance research and nursing science. As another example, it is common that analyses received from a statistician need adjudication of missing data, collapsing of variable categories, communication to fix wrong assumptions, and requests for new or more advanced analyses. Newer nurse researchers may not have a solid background in analyzing data and must be passionate enough about research to seek advice; otherwise, the science produced may have biases and limitations that prevent clinical usefulness and generalizability.

When interviewing nurse researcher candidates, it is important to look for subtle cues that provide evidence of passion. For example, in interviews, we've asked nurse researcher candidates why they had not published any papers (review or research) in recent years. For a few, their responses represented a lack of true passion for advancing nursing science. One responded that she was hoping to get a job that afforded her the time to write at work. When asked why she did not write at home, she stated that she had never thought of it. Another admitted that she had a fear of writing but would begin if she got the job. A passionate nurse researcher will be able to easily discuss collaborative relationships formed and consultative services used to advance nursing science and evidence-based practice.

Moreover, in previous years, nurses who applied for nurse researcher jobs had strong backgrounds in teaching nursing research courses, but very little, or distant, practical research experiences. We've also had doctorate-prepared nurses who verbalized a desire to change careers from academic, clinical, or administration foci to research. The change could be a positive move for the nursing department, nurse researcher, and future mentees; but if the nurse researcher does not display a great deal of passion for clinical research, he or she may not be internally motivated to obtain practical research skills needed to ensure he or she provides strong coaching or mentorship advice that truly advances science. Further, in academic settings, doctorate-prepared nurses may feel entitled (or superior, based on their nursing knowledge and/or skills), and students generally look up to them as leaders. In hospital organizations, previous academic nurses who become nurse researchers will have the best chance of succeeding if they have a modest disposition (Bauer-Wu, Epshtein, & Reid Ponte, 2006). Table 2.3 provides key nurse researcher responsibilities in clinical hospital organizations. Over time, nurse researchers will gain on-the-job research skills, but a low level of passion for research will be displayed by low overall productivity in managing multiple mentee-led research projects, and slow or no growth in developing and managing their own programs of research. Ultimately, fewer nurses will receive the benefit of coaching or mentorship at any given time, reducing potential program outcomes and ultimately reducing the hospital organization's return on investment.

TABLE 2.3 Nurse Researcher Key Responsibilities Within Hospital and Health System Organizations

RESPONSIBILITIES	DETAILS
Increase Research Knowledge	• Nursing research conference planning • Research workshops • Informal 1:1 and group education (related to topics in "serve as a resource")
Forge Collaborations	• With key personnel in other hospital or ambulatory care departments, especially librarians, grant writers, artists, biostatisticians, database analysts, and informatics • With other hospitals and ambulatory care centers • With nursing faculty of academic programs • With doctorate-prepared nurse researchers who have similar job descriptions • With doctorate-prepared nurse researchers who share a similar program of research or clinical specialty • With advanced practice nurses (and those who received clinical-doctorate of nursing practice degrees) interested in conducting or participating in nursing research • With grant funding agencies, nursing organizations, for-profit corporations with investigator-led grant opportunities, and other private or public sector sources, as applicable

(continued)

TABLE 2.3 Nurse Researcher Key Responsibilities Within Hospital and
Health System Organizations (*continued*)

RESPONSIBILITIES	DETAILS
Serve as a Resource	• Answer questions about research question development using PICOTS • In completing a literature review • In determining the best study design • In quantitative and qualitative research methods selection • In institutional review board policies and procedures, research quality, and research compliance (federal regulations) policies and procedures • In study implementation • In ensuring policies and procedures regarding confidentiality of data are maintained • In understanding analyses and meeting analysis needs • In translating findings • In accurate and well formatted oral and poster presentations • In writing, editing, and submitting papers for publication • In generating local and external media attention of research findings and implications • In research accounting • Professional development of nurse researcher colleagues, advanced practice nurses, clinical nurses, and research support staff
Establish Formal Relationships With Academic Facilities	• Adjunct or joint academic or clinical appointments within hospital organization, when applicable • Adjunct academic appointments external to hospital organization, including internationally
Stimulate a Culture of Inquiry	• Guide leadership in establishing and updating internal research structures, systems, and processes that support, nurture, and advance evidence-based nursing practice and research • Develop programs that address barriers to research advancement • Enhance facilitators of research advancement • Reinforce and upgrade research programs based on changing political, social, organizational/administrative and patient care needs • Create resources that stimulate interest in research; e.g., annual internal funding programs, internships and fellowships, grand rounds by external nationally recognized research or clinical experts • Create opportunities for nursing research councils (hospital or unit level) to develop resources; e.g., journal clubs, sacred cow campaigns, and writing workshops
Oversee, Guide, or Informally Lead Research to Support Staff Nurse Mentees	• Address barriers to research start-up and implementation • Work within constraints of operating budget and resources • Connect research nurse coaches/mentees with clinical teams that have available resources; e.g., infection control, education, and quality and patient safety personnel • Provide guidance and implement processes to meet study requirements including eligibility and study parameters when appropriate

PICOTS, population, intervention or indicator, comparator or control, outcome, time, setting.

Second, although a terminal research degree in nursing, education, or science (PhD, DNSc, EdD, ScD) is not absolutely mandatory, there are advantages to hiring nurses with research doctorate degrees. A research doctorate background provides foundational knowledge in research theories, quantitative and qualitative methodologies, and statistical analysis methods. For nurse researchers without terminal research degrees, foundational research knowledge can certainly be gained through practical experiences on the job, self-study, postgraduate college courses, collaboration with external research colleagues, and continuing education classes. Lack of research knowledge may slow productivity, especially if a nurse researcher does not have a network of readily available resources. Some research proposals might contain methodological flaws and biases that create internal and external threats to validity, threats to reliability of findings, a lower level of trust in results, and an inability to disseminate findings in high quality peer-reviewed journals. When nurse mentees learn that data collection was nonessential or that advice given and followed on study methods or analyses was inaccurate, motivation to continue the project and enthusiasm for initiating new research might be dampened. Also, for programs that need to demonstrate research outcomes in a short timeline, a doctorate-prepared nurse researcher with practical research skills has a higher likelihood of meeting goals and deadlines.

Third, nurse researchers' curriculum vitae provide individualized qualities related to productivity, progression in a program of research, and, indirectly, research passion that could enhance (or hinder) research program sustainability. Features to look for are:

(1) The nurse researcher's publication history:

- Escalating review or research publications in recent years (compared to past years) in peer-reviewed journals.
- First author and senior author status (senior author refers here to the last author, who was a coach or mentor to the team) on review or research publications in peer-reviewed journals.
- Co-author status of research publications that include authors representing different professions and multiple sites.

The nurse researcher's publication history is informative for several reasons:

- Peer-review journal publication history provides knowledge about researcher capabilities in working through the peer-review and page-press processes of getting published.
- Peer-review research journal escalation provides information about capability and tenacity in developing and completing research and in seeking out and facilitating interdisciplinary and multisite research.
- Peer-review research topics/paper titles can provide evidence of the depth of research on a concept or in a field of study, the depth of knowledge about analyses used in answering research questions, and even in the strength of

research designs. For example, use of only descriptive statistics and uni-variable or univariate analyses may reflect a lack of depth of understanding of strong analysis methods. If most papers use a qualitative or database design, or used nonvalidated surveys, the nurse researcher may indirectly be demonstrating weaknesses in specific research design or analysis methods that may reduce the potential to produce high quality research.

- Multiple papers with senior author status in a short period of time provide evidence of skills in mentoring/coaching others through the paper-writing process.

(2) Evidence of PI status of investigator-initiated funded studies and external funding from non-profit organizations, government, or for-profit corporations

- Provides evidence of seeking (grant writing), obtaining, and managing external funding, including research accounting.

(3) Active volunteerism in health care working groups, task forces, and committees/councils at a national level.

- Volunteerism provides evidence of leadership, knowledge, teamwork, and a spirit of giving back to the health care community, as national committee work usually involves multidisciplinary experts who come together for mutual purposes.
- Volunteerism enhances mentorship, leadership, confidence in knowledge and skills, awareness of diverse views, and emotional intelligence.
- Volunteerism enlarges our spheres of knowing and influence, and may lead to longstanding relationships that promote new knowledge, services, and resources that are useful to nursing research work.

Finding experienced nurse researchers with these qualities may not be easy, depending on your market environment and academic partnerships. Many nurse researchers grow into their jobs after they complete a research-doctorate degree program. When nurses advance professionally to nurse researcher positions without the benefit of previous research skills and experience, opportunities to shadow experienced nurse researchers in hospital organizations with well-developed nursing research programs should be embraced. If possible, novice nurse researchers should shadow at more than one site to gain experiences in the role responsibilities described in Table 2.3. A fellowship program might allow new nurse researchers to spend weeks or months being embedded in a nursing research program. The fellowship should provide coaching, mentorship, counseling, education, and active participation in multiple aspects of research work (rather than just observation) that enhance understanding of the importance of teamwork, collaboration, vision for the job role, and organizational fit. Classroom education and experiential training of hospital research fundamentals will enhance research nurses' ability to coach and mentor nurses toward successful research project completion, in the face of clinical nurse mentee constraints (primarily time) and research barriers discussed in Chapter 1. Table 2.4 provides a list of fundamental research education themes important to clinical research.

When considering how nurse researchers should use their time in their roles, it is important to consider the scope of work and strategic goals of the nursing department. In a hospital with few nursing employees, the nurse

TABLE 2.4 Fundamental Research Education Themes Important to Clinical Research*

THEMES	SUBTHEMES
Study designs	• Practical, feasible quantitative and qualitative designs • Intent-to-treat principle • Randomization vs. convenience sampling • Observational designs • Longitudinal vs. cross-sectional designs • Using large datasets and electronic medical records • Types of blinding (and ethics of blinding) • Threats to internal and external validity
Protocol development	• Elements of a quantitative and qualitative protocol • Details related to data collection (who are the subjects [if more than one group], what data are collected, where is data collection taking place, when is data collection taking place or what conditions are present, by whom is data being collected) • Details related to protecting data confidentiality • Overcoming expected barriers • Roles and responsibilities of co-investigators • Need for a data safety monitoring board • Timeline after review board approval • Sponsored vs. non-sponsored protocols
Measurement of outcomes	• Valid and reliable methods of assessing outcomes • Investigator developed tools: content validity testing, pre-study initiation and reliability testing in selected sample
Statistics	• Sample size; pilot vs. nonpilot data • Analysis goals: superiority, non-inferiority, or equivalence • Subgroup analyses • Developing sample size and statistical analyses plans
Informed consent	• Elements needed when developing written informed consent and research information sheet documents • Process of informed consent • Documentation of informed consent (when needed; messages) • Research involving children; consent and assent • Vulnerable populations
Recruitment	• Recruitment flyers/advertisements • Recruitment language • Subject compensation • Personnel who can be involved in the process

(continued)

TABLE 2.4 Fundamental Research Education Themes Important to Clinical Research (*continued*)

THEMES	SUBTHEMES
Data collection	• Case report forms format and content • Using electronic databases to collect and store data • Data management (overall) and integrity/quality assessment methods • Dealing with missing data • Ensuring data collection to meet Consolidated Standards of Reporting Trials (CONSORT) checklist and diagram criteria
Protocol deviations and adverse events	• Definitions of unanticipated adverse events and serious adverse events • Definitions of protocol deviations • Reporting requirements
Reporting and publishing research	• The right meeting/conference and journal • Writing a winning abstract and paper
Translating research	• When to translate • Steps of translation, including buy-in from leaders • Sustaining changes in clinical practice once implemented

*Education surrounding research regulations, research quality, and protection of human subjects are discussed in Chapters 5 and 6.

researcher may have a wide range of responsibilities that may expand beyond research. For example, the role may include focus on promoting evidence-based practice, ensuring high quality nursing care, completing administrative projects, and coordinating the hospital's Magnet Recognition Program.® Both a single or multilevel focus can be impactful. In some job descriptions, nurse researchers may be asked to focus solely on coaching or mentoring nurses and not on developing and maintaining their own programs of research. Arguments for a coaching- and mentoring-only roles are part-time work status, limited operational funding for nursing research personnel, and a program goal focused solely on promoting clinical nurse-led research. However, one main negative of job descriptions that do not include nurse researcher responsibilities in managing their own programs of research is that others (within and external to the hospital organization) will believe that practical research skills are lacking, and that the nursing research produced might be lower quality. Since these nurse researchers would not be presenting or publishing their own research, their curriculum vitae related to research would be diminished. Some would say that nurse researchers do not need to "do," they just need to "know" and be able to effectively communicate with mentees. The downside of not "doing" is that nursing departments are constantly evolving. Solutions will be easily recognizable to nurse researchers who are grounded in practical experience. Moreover, "doing" hones skills, especially in writing for publication or grant submission. Federal research rules and policies are applied more practically when researchers understand the practical application of the rules and policies. Volunteer roles on national committees are predicated by expertise that emerges from visibility via published papers and completed research that was nationally funded. Finally, some clinical nurses will relate more closely to nurse researchers who are also principal investigators, as they appreciate being led by example, not just theory.

Nurse researchers must ensure that their programs of research match the strategic boundaries of the hospital organization and nursing department. For example, if a nurse researcher's program of research revolves around prevention of disease, subjects may come from community and senior centers. But, if the job focus is acute care, nursing leadership may not embrace funding time spent in an outpatient wellness program of research. Nurse leadership may not understand the global reach that an individual program of research may have unless individuals involved or their research findings gain national media attention. Nurse leadership may benefit from educational programs or a business plan that includes the benefits of a nursing research program (discussed in Chapter 1) and information about how a specific nursing research program aligns with strategic goals.

Nurse Researcher Performance Expectations

Hospital-based nursing research departments may be costly and generally do not generate income, unless they are linked to academic institutions with large federal funding or receipt of corporate or organizational funding. To provide a return on the investment for hiring doctorate-prepared nurse researchers, objective outcomes should be developed and discussed at hire and in annual performance reviews. Objective outcomes may be based on specific strategic goals of the nursing department and therefore change from year to year, or be clearly defined and stable, to allow nurses to work toward common goals and grow in their roles. At the Cleveland Clinic, we have minimal yearly performance expectations of doctorate-prepared nurse researchers and expect consistent escalation above the minimum expectation level to achieve an exceptional performance review or to advance in job title.

Currently, there are four annual performance expectations that must be achieved and a fifth that is desired. The first expectation is two publications in peer-reviewed journals or books as first author per year. The papers can be review or research focused, but do not count if they are editorials, columns, opinions, or letters to the editor. Papers must be published during the fiscal year to count; a paper that is accepted but not yet published (in press) or published electronically ahead of print would not meet expectations. The purpose is to show that nurse researchers are leaders in advancing research and evidence-based practice through dissemination. A requirement to publish also maintains writing skills and promotes expertise in the field (since a review of literature is most often part of the process).

The second expected outcome is evidence of presenting (oral or poster) as a primary speaker at two national meetings per year. The presentations can be invited or via abstract acceptance. In research or clinical presentations with multiple authors, first author status is required to meet expectations. The rationale behind this expectation is that as nurse researchers increase publications in their program of research, they are more likely to be asked to present at national meetings in their specialty. Writing abstracts and presenting papers maintains and enhances the nurse's presence as an expert, and provides opportunities to meet with colleagues at national meetings and to gain new knowledge and ideas for future research. Further, hospital organizations and nursing departments receive exposure (branding) when the presenter is introduced.

The third expectation is evidence of grant work by writing and submitting grants for self- or mentee-funding to conduct research. Although many research projects are simple enough to be completed with internal funding and resources obtained through the nursing research program, grant funding for clinical nurses may be extremely important, especially when trying to overcome the barrier of time. By making grant work a goal, nurse researchers are reminded to ask nurses about organizations they belong to, assess grant possibilities that match mentored research project themes, and seek support from corporations when federal, state, or organization grants are not available.

The fourth expected outcome is for each nurse researcher to receive "meets" or "exceeds" expectations evaluations from mentees each year. Equally important (and maybe even more important than maintaining a program of research) is to meet the needs of clinical nurse mentees. Our evaluation form was designed by nurse researchers and includes 10 criteria on general working relationships, 11 criteria on specific research projects, and a comment section (Table 2.5 provides the brief wording of the criteria). For criteria items, nurse mentees respond using a Likert-type scale from 1, *unable to rate,* to 5, *exceptional performance.* The process is completed online. Nurse researchers are asked to provide the names of all mentees in the past year. Each name is numbered in alphabetical order and a random number generator is used to randomly select 13 names (with the goal of receiving 10 completed forms). Mentees receive an e-mail request with a link to the evaluation form. Mentees are expected to provide their names on each evaluation form, although nurse researchers only receive a summary of results and comments without mentee names. In addition to annual mentee evaluation of nurse researchers, peer evaluations are an important process of ensuring that nursing research program nurse researchers demonstrate teamwork, partnership, engagement, and cohesiveness. There should be a minimum of four team members evaluating each other before embarking on a peer review process within the program. On our form, collaboration criteria includes four items on congeniality, two items on adaptability, four items on effectiveness, three items on team spirit, and two items on community. Job-related criteria include four items on technical excellence, three items on innovativeness, one ethics item, and two items on teaching/coaching.

TABLE 2.5 Brief Item Content of the Two Criteria Used in Mentee Evaluations of Nurse Researchers

GENERAL WORKING RELATIONSHIPS	SPECIFIC RESEARCH PROJECTS
Positive behaviors	Objective evaluation research processes that lead to improvements in the research plan or mentee understanding of the plan
Pleasantness	
Honesty and truthfulness	Progress toward research goals
Respect of mentee beliefs and values	Responsive to inquiries
Embraces differences of mentees	Timely completion of agreed upon work
Encouragement and support when generating research ideas	Offers assistance
Helps mentee to feel a sense of accomplishment	Clarifies ideas and research questions
	Provides study design recommendations
Flexibility with schedule	Provides study analyses recommendations
Interested in mentee's research goals	Provides writing guidance
Passionate about nursing research	Provides guidance in ethics committee application
	Is resourceful in using software, supplies, and devices

A desired expectation is for nurse researchers to become involved in health care-related volunteer work at the local, regional, state, or national level. Many nurse researchers are reviewers and editorial board members for nursing and biomedical journals. Volunteering to review papers is a wonderful way to altruistically give back to our profession and is appreciated. But more important to the hospital organization, the nursing research department, and nurse researchers themselves is active involvement in policy, practice, standards, performance measures, and clinical, research, or quality initiatives, committees, and task forces led by national organizations. Participation provides nurse researchers with global views on clinical themes of interest, increases their insights of future directions of organizations and legislative and political parties, and connects providers with similar backgrounds and expertise. During volunteer work, nurse researchers' views may be used in developing solutions to problems or in future planning and leadership. Specific to nursing research, insight into patient population research at a national level may be useful in local research planning.

The term "nurse mentee" has been used to describe nurses receiving nurse researcher support. For many nurses, research is like a foreign language; there is a lack of comfort, knowledge, and self-efficacy for research behaviors. Nurse researchers are paid by the nursing department to provide support; many nurses require more than mentorship—they require coaching. Thus, coaching is appropriate and appreciated. If nurse researchers provide coaching

TABLE 2.6 Characteristics of Coaching Versus Mentoring

COACHING REFERS TO TAKING A LEADERSHIP ROLE IN THE *DIRECT* LEARNING AND GROWTH OF OTHERS	MENTORING REFERS TO TAKING A LEADERSHIP ROLE IN *GUIDING* LEARNING AND DEVELOPMENT
Uses practices and strategies to:	**Encourages mentee to:**
• Provide direct teaching and training in technical aspects of new skills • Focus on strengths and overcoming weaknesses • Manage communication to ensure two-way understanding	• Pursue goals with a positive attitude • Examine values, beliefs, and ideals • Be an assertive questioner • Be an attentive listener • Learn through inquiry • Take risks by being an active participant

support (see Table 2.6 for characteristics of coaching and mentoring; Dorval, Isaksen, & Noller, 2001), it is appropriate to be listed on the research proposal as a co-investigator or coach and on presentations and publications as the last (senior) author. However, it is not appropriate to be listed as the first author, no matter the level of support provided, as long as the nurse mentee participated in research processes. Nurses reported that research mentorship was the most important resource available to them (Patterson Kelly, Turner, & Gabel Speroni, 2013). Moreover, when we interviewed clinical nurses before developing our program, they were averse to having nurse researchers "take over" their projects.

Nurse Researcher Job Levels and Escalating Responsibilities

For many professional nursing roles beyond clinical work, there are no professional advancement levels. In hospital organizations, nurse researchers carry many job titles that may include the words director or coordinator, and clinical nurse specialist (Kirkpatrick McLaughlin, Gabel Speroni, Patterson Kelly, Guzzetta, & Desale, 2013) even though, in many cases, they do not have subordinate employees who report to them. In 2004 when the nursing research program was being developed, there were two job titles for nurse researchers, based on academic degree and research skills and outcomes. Recently, we expanded from two to four levels, to increase opportunity for professional advancement among researchers with varying education and training. Research titles and brief descriptions of minimal qualifications for each level are provided in Table 2.7. When nurse researchers are in a solo position, no matter if the job title and description include leadership responsibilities, there is a need to demonstrate a progressive vision for nursing research and the ability to engage others in that vision. Further, the solo nurse researcher must lead and direct initiatives that integrate nursing research into all aspects of nursing practice; serve as the chairperson for nursing research and other professional practice councils; ensure a consistent, structured approach to nursing research (for self and all mentees) that supports the nursing research framework; and promote data-based decision making by developing the skills of departmental nursing leaders.

TABLE 2.7 Nursing Research Program Job Titles and Brief Descriptions

NURSE RESEARCHER JOB TITLE	BRIEF DESCRIPTION	ADVANCEMENT PATH
Nurse Researcher	• Minimum: Master's degree in nursing or related filed (MSN or MN) • Minimum of 3 years of clinical experience as a staff nurse or clinical nurse specialist • Demonstrated advanced skills in human relations, communication, and interdisciplinary collaboration • Publication experience • Research activity may include paper and poster presentation • Knowledge of the extramural grant funding application process • Must be qualified for a faculty appointment with a collegiate school of nursing	• Nurse scientist (if DNP degree) • Senior nurse researcher (if research doctorate degree) • For MSN, no advancement
Nurse Scientist	• Minimum: DNP or other clinical doctorate with evidence of research-based capstone project or research experience • Demonstrated advanced skills in human relations, communication, and interdisciplinary collaboration • Publication experience (research or clinical topics) in nursing journals • Podium presentation experience at local and national meetings is desired • Prefer academic research background that includes multiple research methods, data collection, and database work, even if as an assistant • Minimum of 3 years of clinical experience as a staff nurse, clinical nurse specialist, or clinical faculty • Has knowledge of the extramural grant funding application process • Must be qualified for faculty appointment with a collegiate school of nursing	• For DNP, no advancement
Senior Nurse Researcher	• Research doctorate in nursing (PhD or DNSc) or related field (ScD, EdD, etc.) with completed research dissertation • Publication experience related to research activity, and presentation experience (paper or poster) • Minimum of 3 years of research experience including experience with experimental design, multiple methodologies, databases, and data analysis software • Must be qualified for faculty appointment with a collegiate school of nursing; upon employment, maintains faculty appointment	• Senior nurse scientist

(continued)

TABLE 2.7 Nursing Research Program Job Titles and Brief Descriptions (*continued*)

NURSE RESEARCHER JOB TITLE	BRIEF DESCRIPTION	ADVANCEMENT PATH
Senior Nurse Scientist	• Research doctorate in nursing (PhD or DNSc) or related field (ScD, EdD, etc.) with completed research dissertation; • Minimum of 3 years of research experience, with extensive experience with multiple experimental and qualitative designs, multiple methodologies, databases, and data analysis software • Experience in extramural grant funding application and in managing funds • Demonstrated expertise in interpersonal relationships, and educative and consultative roles • Escalating publication experience of research activities in peer-reviewed journals • Minimum of 5 years of clinical experience as a staff nurse, clinical nurse specialist, or clinical faculty • Must be qualified for faculty appointment with a collegiate school of nursing	• No advancement
All positions	• Be able to multitask, be flexible in assignments, be results/outcomes-driven and work collaboratively • Within scope of job, requires critical thinking skills, decisive judgment, and the ability to work with minimal supervision • Must be able to work in a stressful environment	• Not applicable

DNP, doctorate of nursing practice; MN, master of nursing; MSN, master of nursing science.

Nurse Researcher Scope

Papers in the literature discuss building nursing research programs in hospitals or other practice settings (Jeffs, Smith, Beswick, Maoine, & Ferris, 2013; Kirkpatrick McLaughlin et al., 2013; Patterson Kelly et al., 2013) and in one research report, investigators described research program requirements (Kirkpatrick McLaughlin et al., 2013); however, no reports other than a paper authored by my colleague and I (Albert & Siedlecki 2008) reported the capacity of one nurse researcher. It may be that hospitals with nursing research programs limit the number of nurse-led research studies initiated per year, and nurse researchers never reach work capacity. When research program scholarly outcomes were collected from 160 United States hospitals, the average number of studies initiated per year was 3.76 and ranged from 1.95 in hospitals with less than 100 beds to 6.4 studies in hospitals with greater than 1,000 beds (Kirkpatrick McLaughlin et al., 2013). In our nursing research program, one full time equivalent nurse researcher handles approximately 22 to 35 active research projects at any given time, including both his or her own and those of mentees. Funded studies and randomized controlled, multisite, and longitudinal designs can be more time intensive, especially when they are led by a mentee, rather than a nurse researcher, and require closer follow-up by the research coach/mentor. One factor affecting capacity is the number of employees who are students working on graduate degrees. Nurse researchers are assigned to students who are in the final project (doctorate of nursing practice) or dissertation (philosophy doctorate) phase of graduate school requirements to ensure that what is submitted to the institutional review board for oversight is scientifically sound, ethical, and feasible. Often, revisions are needed. Nurse researchers want to be sure that the grade earned by students represents the students' own work, not that of the nurse researcher; therefore, revisions may take more time to complete. Other factors affecting research project capacity per nurse researcher are time spent in nursing research program meetings, classes, and professional growth opportunities; the scope of office project work to be completed, such as preparing educational presentations, planning research conferences, and presence at council and committee meetings; and the scope of nursing department or hospital project commitments. Since research work is very time consuming and may require blocks of time to make progress, nurse researchers must protect their time to ensure essential work is completed.

VOICES OF NURSE RESEARCHERS

Karen L. Rice, DNS, APRN, ACNS-BC, ANP
Director, The Center for Nursing Research, Ochsner Health System, New Orleans, Louisiana

Shelley S. Thibeau, PhD, RN-NIC
Senior RN Researcher, The Center for Nursing Research, Ochsner Health System, New Orleans, Louisiana

Although Ochsner Health System does not establish a goal for the number of research studies conducted each year, integration of the Iowa Model in the council and unit-based structures serves as a pipeline for evidence-based practice (EBP) projects that generate researchable questions. Since 2006, the flagship hospital at our Magnet® facility conducted six to 10 research studies each year. Studies included those led by two dedicated nurse scientists, and by clinical nurse specialists, nurse practitioners, hospital nurses, external nurse researchers, and nurses completing studies for academic requirements (i.e., master's and doctoral degrees).

Nurse Researchers in Academic–Practice Partnerships

Dedicated, doctorate-prepared nurse researchers are an essential foundational element to building and nurturing a hospital nursing research program. But personnel are the largest cost of any program and hospital size may preclude the ability to hire a full-time nurse researcher, especially during program construction and start-up, when research volume is low. Further, an academic hospital may already have a strategic relationship in place with a university/college/ school of nursing for nursing education and professional development or may be willing to develop an academic partnership with a local university/college.

For some nursing leaders, developing a strategic alliance or partnership with an academic setting to provide nurse researcher support is a means to minimize program costs and provide experienced nurse researchers to coach or mentor nurses in research (Boland, Kamikawa, Inouye, Latimer, & Marshall, 2010; Rao, Rich, & Meleis, 2014). However, when cross-institutional collaborations were studied, collegiate participants had different perceptions of accessibility of resources than practice setting participants. Of note, perceptions of accessibility to grant development, informatics, and supportive personnel (research assistants who completed day-to-day activities) were lower among practice settings; and both groups had concerns about conflicts of interest (Tubbs-Cooley, Martsolf, Pickler, Morrison, & Wardlaw, 2013). Thus, effective academic–practice partnerships in nursing research can strengthen evidence-based nursing practice, but systems and processes may need to be implemented to ensure that hospital nurses are adequately supported.

VOICES OF NURSE RESEARCHERS

Karen L. Rice, DNS, APRN, ACNS-BC, ANP
Director, The Center for Nursing Research, Ochsner Health System, New Orleans, Louisiana

Shelley S. Thibeau, PhD, RN-NIC
Senior RN Researcher, The Center for Nursing Research, Ochsner Health System, New Orleans, Louisiana

The single most important infrastructure resource to a successful nursing research program at our facility is having a dedicated nursing research department, led by a doctorate-prepared nurse scientist. Having an experienced, dedicated nurse scientist is essential to rally appropriate resources, mentor staff at all levels of expertise, and facilitate entry of external researchers to conduct

(continued)

VOICES OF NURSE RESEARCHERS (*continued*)

research at our facility. In addition, this type of infrastructure fosters opportunities to engage in national collaborative nursing and interprofessional research studies, and positions the institution to compete for extramural funding.

INTRANET RESOURCES

Nurses need research resources to overcome barriers in using research evidence and conducting research. The focus of Chapter 3 is on resources that aid the success of nursing research programs. The focus here is on one resource that is foundational to success: a well-developed internal (intranet) website. Our nursing research center intranet site is grouped into seven segments (see Table 2.8). Intranet site information should be based on users' needs, and since users are generally nurses who are novice researchers, the site must be organized and labeled so that nurses can find information easily. Figures 2.2 to 2.5 provide page 1 of the content of three templates and one checklist available on our website. Figure 2.6 provides the Cleveland Clinic Evidence-Based Practice Model. Templates are an important resource since they simplify work and create uniformity. Checklists help nurses stay organized and ensure they meet all requirements or department expectations. How-to

TABLE 2.8 Intranet Research Resources

INTRANET SECTION HEADERS	MATERIALS INCLUDED

General Information	• Templates (three of 13 examples are listed below and in Figures 2.2–2.4)
	  ▪ Quantitative clinical research proposal
	  ▪ Content validity index testing
	  ▪ Example data collection form
	• Checklists (one of 8 examples is listed below and in Figure 2.5)
	  ▪ Protocol Feasibility Checklist
	• Evidence-based practice
	• Cleveland Clinic NI evidence-based practice model (Figure 2.6)
	  ▪ Cleveland Clinic NI strength of evidence model
	  ▪ Cleveland Clinic NI quality of evidence model
	  ▪ Cleveland Clinic NI rapid appraisal tool
	• Research versus quality versus product evaluation
	  ▪ Handouts that differentiate the three themes
	• Contacts
	  ▪ Nursing research program organizational chart
	  ▪ Picture of team members with contact information

(*continued*)

TABLE 2.8 Intranet Research Resources (*continued*)

INTRANET SECTION HEADERS	MATERIALS INCLUDED

Conducting Research	• Overview
	  ▪ Handout on developing a research question
	  ▪ Handout on the steps of the nursing research process
	• Literature review
	  ▪ Handouts on how to review qualitative and quantitative papers
	  ▪ Handout on conducting a literature review and creating a summary (synthesis) document
	• Writing a proposal
	  ▪ Templates for quantitative and qualitative proposals
	• Resources
	  ▪ Common issues associated with research studies
	  ▪ Table of research terms and statistics definitions

Disseminating Research and Evidence-Based Practice	• Creating posters
	  ▪ Poster board presentation template
	  ▪ Tabletop poster template
	• Completed posters
	  ▪ PDFs of completed nursing research posters, since 2010
	  ▪ Listed by first author's last name, year, and title
	• Completed literature reviews of current evidence on a topic
	  ▪ PDFs of completed syntheses of literature reviews on specific concepts, since 2013; listed by first author's last name, year and title

Education, Policies, Grant Funding, and Councils	• Students: Contains seven documents (forms, checklists, overview sheet, and mandatory education requirements) needed to conduct research as a student • Education: Contains research education instructions, handouts, quizzes, and a list of nurses who completed all requirements • NuRF Award*: Instructions, application, and other forms • NuRF Lit Award*: Instructions, application, and other forms • Policies: Three nursing department policies and multiple nursing research program standards of practice • Councils: Links to Nursing Research Councils
References on Research	• Documents that provide references on instrument development, sample size, using visual analog scales, and different analysis methodologies
Institutional Review Board	• Review board documents of high interest to nurses: common issues associated with research studies and frequently asked questions
Useful Links	• Twelve internal and external links of resources that include the American Nurses Association Research toolkit, the Virginia Henderson Global Nursing e-Repository, a random number generator, nursing organization links, nursing journal links, and more

*Described in Chapter 3.

Note: To purchase Cleveland Clinic nursing research resources (tools, templates, and instructions), go to www.onadeo.com

NI, Nursing Institute.

Cleveland Clinic Quantitative Nursing Research Proposal Template
Format and Content

Title/Investigators/Version Number
Title should reflect the question (topic) you are addressing. Place on a separate page. Keep as short as possible.

Investigators: Include yourself and ALL other collaborators. First name listed is assumed to be the Principal Investigator (PI). Include your nursing research mentor as well (can place "mentor" in parentheses, as desired).

Version number: Place the version of your proposal in a footnote. Generally, version 1 is the version that the institutional review board (IRB) receives for approval. Anytime you make a change and submit an amendment to the IRB due to protocol revision, the version number is updated.

Abstract
250 words that provide an overview of the problem, study methods, data collection methods, sample characteristics, and sample size.
   Place the abstract on a separate page.

Background/Review of Literature/Significance
Briefly state the background; summarize the literature—what is unknown or what is controversial, or the current state of knowledge to indicate why a study is needed. Include key references. When applicable, include how your research is significant to nursing.

Purpose, Specific Aims and/or Research Questions
Clearly state the purpose of your study (global statement). Then state either the specific aim(s) [statement(s) that include(s) the outcomes or endpoints you wish to learn about], research question(s) or hypothesis(es).
   The research purpose and aim, research questions, or hypotheses must be well formulated; this section is the single most important ingredient for success.

Methodology
(a)   Study Group Definition/Subjects
Who are the subjects? What is the study group that is pertinent to your research question? Define both inclusion and exclusion criteria and the inclusive dates, and justify these.
   Comparison Group/Denominator: If you propose that something is improved or different, ask *"Then what?"* You need a comparison group. If you propose to study an *event*, this is a numerator; you need *both numerator and denominator.*

FIGURE 2.2 Quantitative research proposal template.
Adapted from Albert and the Office of Nursing Research and Innovation, Cleveland Clinic (2006).

handouts provide step-by-step instructions and references that provide guidance and support. External links to important research, publications, and nursing organization sites and resources help broaden knowledge, provide new perspectives, save time, and facilitate research work. A sample case report form provides guidance in how to develop one so that it is aesthetically appealing, professional looking (uses white space, italics, bold font, and shading to separate sections, creates emphasis and easy readability), and easily understood.

Intranet sites should be used for more than just procuring information. Having a section devoted to research results (e.g., PDFs of research posters), research awards, and stories of nurse accomplishments in advancing nursing

Content Validity Index for [place title of survey here] Survey

About yourself: Are you a(n): ☐ NM or ANM ☐ CI or CNS ☐ Staff nurse

How long have you worked on your present unit? _____ years.

For each of the statements in the survey below, please assess content validity by providing information about:

Item relevance (does the statement belong on a survey of assessment of [place theme of survey here]), clarity, and importance

CONTENT RELEVANCE	ITEM CLARITY	ITEM IMPORTANCE
1. Item is not relevant 2. Unable to assess relevance without item revision 3. Relevant but needs minor alteration 4. Item is very relevant and succinct	1. Unclear 2. Unclear without revision 3. Clear with minor alteration 4. Clear	1. Not important; remove 2. Somewhat important; keep on survey if room 3. Important; keep on survey 4. Very important; do not remove from survey

Choose a number for each statement:	Content Relevance Score (1–4)	Item Clarity Score (1–4)	Item Importance Score (1–4)

FIGURE 2.3 Content Validity Testing Template.
Adapted from Albert and the Office of Nursing Research and Innovation, Cleveland Clinic (2008).

[TITLE] Case Report Form (Template)

Instructions:..
....

General Information
Allied health professional name: Physician name:

Specialty: Specialty:
Hospital: Phone:
City: Fax:
State: e-mail:

Date completing this form: _____

Patient Information
Patient Initials: _____   Gender: ☐ Male   ☐ Female   Age: _____

Ethnic Origin: ☐ African American   ☐ Asian American
                ☐ Caucasian   ☐ Hispanic/Latino/Spanish
                ☐ Native Indian/Alaska Native   ☐ Other (*please specify*): _____

Cardiovascular Status
CURRENT cardiovascular disease (*check all that apply*)
☐ Coronary artery disease   ☐ Peripheral vascular disease
☐ Hypertension   ☐ CVA (cerebrovascular accident): Date(s): _____
☐ Myocardial infarction(s): Date(s): _____
☐ Hyperlipidemia
☐ Valvular heart disease (please specify): _____
☐ Other (please specify): _____

PRIOR cardiac INTERVENTION (*check all that apply*)
☐ None
☐ Ablation   Date of most recent (Month, Year): _____
☐ Angioplasty/stent   Date of most recent (Month, Year): _____ No. of vessels: ___
                        Date of most recent (Month, Year): _____ No. of vessels: ___

☐ Coronary artery bypass graft
☐ Repair/correction of congenital abnormality
(please specify): _____

☐ Valves replaced / repaired

FIGURE 2.4 Case Report Form Template.
Adapted from Albert (2008).

science, synthesizing evidence on concepts, and translating evidence into clinical practice personalizes the site and provides evidence that research is doable and important.

NURSING RESEARCH DEPARTMENT DATABASE

To provide a vision of how a nursing research department database could benefit nurses, nurse leaders, and nurse researchers, consider this scenario. A nurse who is a novice to nursing research approaches you for assistance on a

Cleveland Clinic
Office of Nursing Research and Innovation
Protocol Feasibility Checklist

1. Sponsor/Clinical Research Organization (CRO)

Yes No

❏	❏	Has your previous experience with this sponsor/CRO been satisfactory?
❏	❏	If you have had no previous experience with this sponsor/CRO, have you checked the sponsor's/CRO's reputation with colleagues?

2. Population

Yes No

❏	❏	Do you have access to the right patient population?
❏	❏	Will you need to recruit patients from external sources? If so, do you have a plan to do this? Do you have time to do this? Will sponsor provide funding?
❏	❏	Is the proposed enrollment goal realistic? If appropriate, have you performed a power analysis to ensure that you have an adequate sample size?
❏	❏	Is the proposed enrollment period realistic?
❏	❏	Will enrollment compete with other studies seeking the same patients?
❏	❏	Are inclusion/exclusion criteria overly restrictive?
❏	❏	Are vulnerable populations involved, e.g., employees, children, impaired adults with special consent issues?
❏	❏	Do you expect any adverse events or problems that result from research procedures?

3. Protocol

Yes No

❏	❏	Is the protocol well designed?
❏	❏	Is the protocol ethical? Will the IRB have concerns with it?
❏	❏	Is the study question or specific aim important to nurses or nursing practice?
❏	❏	Will the subjects benefit from participating in the study?
❏	❏	Are there risks for subjects who participate in the study? If so, how will you address the risks?
❏	❏	If you do not think the protocol is feasible as written, is the sponsor willing to consider or suggest modifications?
❏	❏	Will coordination with other departments/services be required for study visits or procedures?
❏	❏	Can other services (e.g., lab, radiology) meet the protocol requirements?
❏	❏	Are necessary supplies or equipment available? If not, will the sponsor provide?
❏	❏	Is the study unusually long in duration? (Drop-outs are more likely in long studies.)
❏	❏	If an inpatient study, will floor staff need to be involved?
❏	❏	Are patient compliance problems likely? If so, will it be necessary to monitor subjects' compliance with time-consuming phone calls or mailings of follow-up surveys?
❏	❏	Are all the protocol required parameters captured in the Case Report Form?
❏	❏	Are all the protocol parameters captured in source documents? If not, how will you provide source documentation _____

FIGURE 2.5 Protocol Feasibility Checklist.
Adapted from the Office of Nursing Research and Innovation, Cleveland Clinic (2014).

research study involving massage therapy in orthopedic patients. You do not know of any recent studies by nurses in your hospital on this topic, but in a literature review, a paper was found from your hospital organization. You do not know the nurse investigators personally, as their patient population is not in your area of expertise, and upon a search, you learn that the nurses no longer work at the hospital and the e-mail address for the corresponding author no longer applies. The study design was strong and research methods seemed

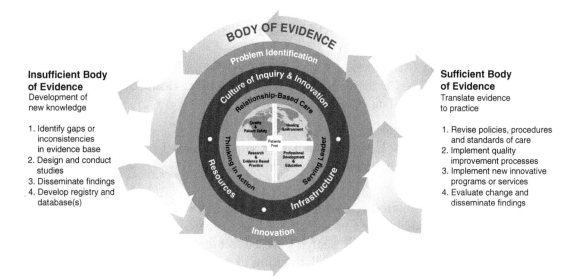

**Insufficient Body
of Evidence**
Development of
new knowledge

1. Identify gaps or
   inconsistencies
   in evidence base
2. Design and conduct
   studies
3. Disseminate findings
4. Develop registry and
   database(s)

**Sufficient Body
of Evidence**
Translate evidence
to practice

1. Revise policies, procedures
   and standards of care
2. Implement quality
   improvement processes
3. Implement new innovative
   programs or services
4. Evaluate change and
   disseminate findings

FIGURE 2.6 Cleveland Clinic Evidence-Based Practice Model.
Adapted from Albert and Siedlecki (2010).

adequate, yet the results were negative for all outcomes. What if you had a research database and (a) found an accessible study protocol, (b) had access to the data analysis to learn about unreported study limitations, and (c) learned that a behind-the-scenes statistician still worked at the hospital?

In another scenario, a chief nursing officer from a smaller hospital in a large health system hears about ongoing nursing research at leadership meetings but wants to see how her hospital compares with others in the system and how fast each project is progressing. What if you had a research database and could (a) view total research projects by hospital, patient populations, nurse investigators, and nurse researcher coaches/mentors, (b) determine the status of each project from a master screen, and (c) find other projects on the same topics after searching by key words?

A research database is a valuable resource for internal tracking of nursing research projects and maintaining statistics, but more important, it can be used as a resource for nurses who lead research and nurse leaders who want to maintain a history of previous and current research, especially since some studies get abandoned, and not all completed research studies get disseminated. A database archives new and emerging knowledge, and is not affected by nurse retirements and terminations. The database provides a wealth of study information that can be used by others conducting research on the same or similar concepts. Without a database or other central repository, individual research project proposal materials, electronic communication, analyses, and other information are maintained on individual computers and are subject to loss.

VOICES OF NURSE RESEARCHERS

Karen L. Rice, DNS, APRN, ACNS-BC, ANP
Director, The Center for Nursing Research, Ochsner Health System,
New Orleans, Louisiana

Shelley S. Thibeau, PhD, RN-NIC
Senior RN Researcher, The Center for Nursing Research,
Ochsner Health System, New Orleans, Louisiana

Research-related activities are tracked using an Excel spreadsheet
maintained by the Center for Nursing Research. Since the
Center for Nursing Research oversees all research and chairs the
Nursing Research Council, tracking of research-related activities
is easily accomplished. Information includes: title of study,
investigators and affiliations, date approved or not approved
by the Nursing Research Council, date approved by the internal
review board (IRB) including type of determination (e.g., exempt,
expedited approval, full panel), date the study was opened, date
the study was closed, type of design (e.g., quantitative, qualitative,
mixed methods), and comments (e.g., single site, multiple site collaborative). In addition, dissemination of research (e.g., podium,
poster, and publications) is also tracked.

Mary Ann Friesen, PhD, RN, CPHQ
Nursing Research and Evidence-Based Practice Coordinator,
Inova Health System, Falls Church, Virginia

Colleen Brooks, BS
Nursing Policy Coordinator Nursing Research and Evidence-Based
Practice Coordinator, Inova Loudoun Hospital, Falls Church, Virginia

One of the challenges for our Nursing Research and Evidence-Based
Practice Council is coordinating and communicating research
studies and EBP activities across a multihospital system. Working
with Information Technology, a database was created that allows
tracking of research studies from proposal through dissemination.
The database allows information to be shared across the system in
a user-friendly manner, and individual reports can be generated to
provide information needed for each hospital. A monthly report is
presented at the system and hospital research and EBP council

(continued)

VOICES OF NURSE RESEARCHERS (*continued*)

meetings so that nurses at each hospital can quickly review the reports to learn what others are doing. The report has helped provide a catalyst for collaboration across hospitals on various research studies.

REFERENCES

Albert, N. M. (2008). *Case report form template*. Cleveland, OH: Cleveland Clinic Foundation.

Albert, N. M., & The Office of Nursing Research and Innovation, Cleveland Clinic. (2006). *Quantitative research proposal template*. Cleveland, OH: Cleveland Clinic Foundation.

Albert, N. M., & The Office of Nursing Research and Innovation, Cleveland Clinic. (2008). *Content validity testing template*. Cleveland, OH: Cleveland Clinic Foundation.

Albert, N. M., & Siedlecki, S. L. (2008). Developing and implementing a nursing research team in a clinical setting. *Journal of Nursing Administration, 38*(2), 90–96.

Albert, N. M., & Siedlecki, S. L. (2010). *Cleveland Clinic evidence based practice model*. Cleveland, OH: Cleveland Clinic Foundation.

Bauer-Wu, S., Epshtein, A., & Reid Ponte, P. (2006). Promoting excellence in nursing research and scholarship in the clinical setting. *Journal of Nursing Administration, 36*(5), 224–227.

Boland, M. G., Kamikawa, C., Inouye, J., Latimer, R. W., & Marshall, S. (2010). Partnership to build research capacity. *Nursing Economics, 28*(5), 314–321, 336.

Dorval, K. B., Isaksen, S. G., & Noller, R. B. (2001). Leadership for learning: Tips for effective mentoring and coaching. In Ken McCluskey (Ed.), *Mentoring for Talent Development*, (pp. 25–36). Lennox, SD: Reclaiming Youth.

Jeffs, L., Smith, O., Beswick, S., Maoine, M., & Ferris, E. (2013). Investing in nursing research in practice settings: A blueprint for building capacity. *Nursing Leadership, 26*(4), 44–59.

Kirkpatrick McLaughlin, M., Gabel Speroni, K., Patterson Kelly, K., Guzzetta, C. E., & Desale, S. (2013). National survey of hospital nursing research, part 1: Research requirements and outcomes. *Journal of Nursing Administration, 43*(1), 10–17.

The Office of Nursing Research and Innovation, Cleveland Clinic. (2014). *Protocol feasibility checklist*. Cleveland, OH: Cleveland Clinic Foundation.

Patterson Kelly, K., Turner, A., & Gabel Speroni, K. (2013). National survey of hospital nursing research, part 2: Facilitators and hindrances. *Journal of Nursing Administration, 43*(1), 18–23.

Rao, A. D., Rich, V. L., & Meleis, A. (2014). A 12-year look back: The University of Pennsylvania nursing academic-practice partnership. *Nurse Leader, 12*(4), 43–47.

Tubbs-Cooley, H. L., Martsolf, D. S., Pickler, R. H., Morrison, C. F., & Wardlaw, C. E. (2013). Development of a regional nursing research partnership for academic and practice collaborations. *Nursing Research and Practice, 2013.* doi: 10.1155/2013/473864

Sandra L. Siedlecki

3

BUILDING BLOCKS FOR A STRONG NURSING RESEARCH PROGRAM

Primary adjuncts to a thriving nursing research program and productive nursing research staff are personnel and resources dedicated to research activities (Albert & Siedlecki, 2008; McLaughlin, Speroni, Kelly, Guzzetta, & Desale, 2013). A nursing research program, big or small, will require sufficient resources to ensure initial success and promote growth and success that is measured by the number of nursing research studies the program generates and supports each year. The larger the hospital organization and the more nurses employed, the more resources will be needed to support research activities. To determine the number of potential nurses involved in research activities at any one time, a good rule of thumb when resources are sufficient, is to expect about 2.5% of nursing employees (2.5 nurses per 100 employees, no matter their roles) to be research nurse investigators or co-investigators in active research studies and another 2.5% (2.5 nurses per 100 employees) to be developing research studies that may or may not succeed to institutional review board (IRB) approval and implementation. A hospital with a nursing staff of 500 nurses will need a plan to support 25 nurses who desire to conduct nursing research, individually or in team projects, at any given time. This chapter provides an overview of nursing research program resources that are building blocks for strong programs that nurture and support the many aspects of research.

PERSONNEL

The most critical and most expensive resource required for a successful nursing research program is personnel. Personnel includes both nursing professionals and ancillary staff. The larger the hospital organization, the greater the need for more than one doctorate-prepared nurse researcher, assuming that nursing research activities are supported without restrictions in size and scope.

For example, some research programs only allow nurses to use validated research tools in the literature, as they do not have nurse researchers with expertise in tool development and psychometric testing. Others only allow quantitative descriptive research designs or qualitative narrative projects as they cannot support the rigor of other research designs that require specific research expertise and ancillary staff.

Nurse Researchers

The cornerstone of a nursing research program is nurse researchers who anchor the program and set the tone for all future growth and development. Lack of research mentors and other supportive services were a major barrier to research production by clinical nurses (Loke, Laurenson, & Wai Lee, 2014; McLaughlin et al., 2013). Thus, it is important that the nursing research program employs the services of nurse research mentors who have sufficient knowledge and experience to mentor novice nurses from identification of a researchable problem to publication and presentation of research findings. Nurse research mentors should be proficient in different research methods and designs and be able to guide nurses through basic design and analysis issues; refer to Chapter 2 for more details. The right number of nurse researcher mentors will prevent delays in meeting with mentees, as delays in meeting regularly may lead to loss of interest in research and potential loss of answers to innovative and interesting research questions.

Supportive and Ancillary Personnel

After nurse researchers are hired, it will be necessary to provide additional supportive and ancillary personnel to assist with research work. The need for supportive and ancillary personnel will depend upon the scope of the nursing research program, the number and type of nursing research studies supported at any given time, and the need to support nursing department goals and objectives. For small programs with a single nurse researcher, minimal nursing supportive personnel are needed but ancillary support, for example, an administrative assistant, statistician, and librarian, may provide valuable support. As the number of studies becomes substantial, or if grant support is received, nurses who can assist with data collection and research accounting will become more important.

Research Nurse Support
A research nurse is a registered nurse trained in IRB policies, procedures, and application processes, study subject recruitment, enrollment and data collection, and database work. Research nurses can develop informed consent

documents, complete website work for IRB submission, yearly renewal, and proposal amendments. They can assess and enroll patients in studies, collect data, develop and use databases, assess the quality of data entered, and clean data, all of which are the most time intensive parts of the nursing research process. For projects that would not be feasible without data collection support, this resource is critical. However, data collection support does not have to be expensive. Research nurse options for IRB, study subject, and database support include hiring full- or part-time temporary nurses (who work when external funding is available) or, for data collection alone, using graduate students from local universities in exchange for a mentored nursing research practicum (refer to Chapter 7 for more details). For funded studies, nursing personnel costs should be included in the budget. Table 3.1 provides considerations when planning costs for nurse personnel for funded studies.

Administrative Assistant Services
As with nursing personnel, the need for an administrative assistant will depend upon the size and scope of the nursing research program and number of studies being supported. A single nurse researcher with five or fewer studies may only require occasional administrative support; however, as the number of

TABLE 3.1 Cost Considerations for Budgeting Research Nurses

COST CATEGORY	CONSIDERATIONS
Basic research work (productive time)	• If the nurse has not already been selected, budget at the highest pay rate in the pay range and consider the length of the research study, as an annual or merit raise may need to be added for each year beyond year one of the study • Include time to get from desk area to clinical research work area when considering costs • Include the costs of delays in enrolling patients, prolonged data collection due to patients who require nurses to read questionnaire items, do not answer the telephone, and other issues ▪ Suggest a minimum of doubling the time needed to collect data required and, if the study is longitudinal or has complex data collection, tripling the amount of time needed from what you estimate.
Education costs (in nonproductive time)	• Include costs of nurse completion of mandatory research and human subjects education at hire • Include costs of ongoing nurse education to meet continuing education requirements for license renewal • Include costs of time spent in nonproductive education associated with nursing research program functions (e.g., an annual nursing research conference)
Fringe costs	• Hospital organization set costs for nonproductive time
Overhead costs	• Hospital organization set costs for administrative time and facilities overhead (lighting, telephone, computer, and other support space and services)

studies and the number of nurse researchers increases, the need for support will also increase, especially if the nursing research program supports graduate students completing research practica or theses, final projects, or dissertations. Criteria for this position would be excellent computer and organizational skills, including knowledge of multiple software programs (Microsoft Word, Excel, Access, Publisher, and Visio programs and IBM's Statistical Package for Social Sciences [SPSS] or other software for statistical analysis), highly flexible with workload, and able to deal with multiple interruptions.

Biostatistician and Statistical Programmer
Even with well-qualified doctorate-prepared nurse researchers, there remains a need for statistical consultation. Ideally, a statistician should be consulted at the beginning of proposal development to assist researchers to develop the sample size and analysis plans. In small nursing research programs, statistical consultation may not be available as a hospital service and consultation with external statisticians may be expensive. Cost for statistical consultation averages about $115 per hour in communities with Midwest economic costs. Statistical programmers are master's and doctorate prepared and complete preparation for analysis, including recoding, transformations, grouping of data, and other functions. Their skill set is different than a statistician's, but costs are the same. Nursing research program costs need to include yearly costs for statistical analysis. Not all nursing research studies require a high level of data analysis. Nurse researchers should have basic knowledge and skill in simple data analysis, such as descriptive and correlational statistics, independent t-test, paired t-test, analysis of variance, and regression.

FUNDING

Leaders of nursing research programs must consider the costs involved in maintenance and growth. The primary costs are associated with personnel (nurse researchers and supportive and ancillary staff) salaries. However, the nursing research program also requires general office space and equipment/ services (printers, computers, software, telephone, and teleconferencing capabilities), general office supplies, travel costs, book costs, and maintenance fees associated with statistical software programs. In addition, programs that include annual nursing research conferences, educational workshops, and funding of programs that support nursing research need adequate funding in order to succeed.

Because of the Health Insurance Portability and Accountability Act (HIPAA) rules, considerations for privacy of data may mean costs for locking filing cabinets and briefcases, using computers that can only be accessed by one person or require password entry, encrypted USB drives and personal computers, space with four walls and doors with locks or high privacy panels, and an external door to the area that locks. In addition to nurse researcher space, special space may be needed for corporate sponsors who visit the hospital to review the research progress of funded studies. They cannot have access to a computer with hospital data and must complete their visitation work in a place that provides privacy and access to materials needed. Finally, as research is often conducted among teams, a conference room is needed if office space is small, to accommodate three to five people, and must have a computer, screen, and teleconferencing capabilities.

Research Program Funding and Support

Funding for a nursing research program will be included in the operating budget of a hospital organization's nursing department. For hospitals that do not have a separate nursing research department, funds are usually placed in a professional development/education, quality, or administrative cost center. Ideally, the nursing research program should have its own operating budget, even if small, so that program costs are not diverted to larger programs with competing needs. A nursing research program can only grow and flourish if it is important enough to stand alone. When there are divided loyalties or sharing of scarce resources, nursing research programs may flounder since many administrators have never completed research and do not understand the need for infrastructure and resources. When nursing research is a priority and is associated with strategic nursing department goals, the research program will grow. Once a nursing research program is developed, it is important that nurse researchers identify internal and external sources of funding to support the conduct of research developed by clinical nurses.

Internal Funding
Internal funding sources are funds made available by the institution to support individual research studies. Many internal funding programs support "release time" for nurses to complete a literature review or research studies. The criteria of the Cleveland Clinic funding mechanisms are described in Table 3.2 and an internship program is described in Chapter 7. When internal funds are available, nurses should submit a research proposal and compete for available funds. In that way, funding is given to projects that are well written, of high quality, scientifically sound, ethical, and feasible.

When considering the distribution of internal funds to support a research study by clinical nurses, it is important that nurses understand that funding is dependent not only on completion of research processes and analyses and presentation at a meeting, but also on publication of study results and translation of findings into practice, when applicable. In this way, scarce resources are appropriately expended for research studies that add to nursing's knowledge base and contribute to improved nursing practice.

TABLE 3.2 Cleveland Clinic Internal Funding Programs

PROGRAM CRITERIA AND EXPECTED OUTCOMES	FREQUENCY	COMPETITIVE	FUNDING LIMIT	NUMBER AVAILABLE
Nursing Research Fund (NuRF) Grant Award • Nursing research study • Well-written proposal that conforms to stated proposal requirements • Nurse as principal investigator • Reasonable and justified budget • Sound methodology • Feasible within financial and time constraints (2 years) • Funding given to the unit where the nurse works; to cover release time and supplies used. Up to $750 may be used for travel • <u>Outcome</u>: Submission of completed research findings to a peer-reviewed journal for publication	Two rounds: Spring and fall	Proposals are peer reviewed. Reviewers are nurse researchers and clinical nurse members of research councils	$2,500 per project; $7,500 per funding period; $15,000 per year	Minimum of three per funding period if each receives maximum funding. More than three if less than the maximum funding used for each
Nursing Research Literature Review (NuRF-LIT) Grant • Literature review of a topic of clinical importance; must provide rationale in application • Hourly nurses (exempt status nurses are not eligible) • Clarity of application • Sound research question • Significant to nursing practice • Funding is given to the nursing unit, not to the nurse completing the literature review; to cover approximately 16 hours of release time • <u>Outcome</u>: Poster showing synthesis of the literature, nursing implications, and clinical practice recommendations based on the evidence presented. Must present findings at a local unit meeting	Two rounds: Spring and fall	Proposals are peer reviewed: See members above	$500 per project; $3,000 per funding period; $6,000 per year	Six per round; 12 per year

External Funding

External funding consists of grant funding from entities outside the hospital organization (see Table 3.3). Previous experience of nurse researchers in obtaining external funding is a critical asset to the nursing research program. Nurse researchers should be well versed in the availability and requirements for submitting grant proposals for consideration for external funding. External funding can be used to provide funds to cover time for the principal investigator and for the cost of supplies, data collection, data entry, data analysis, and in some cases dissemination. In general, there are four basic types of external funding available for nursing research: governmental, professional nursing organization, specialty nursing organization sponsored grants, and corporate funding.

Governmental supported programs, such as the Agency for Healthcare Research and Quality (AHRQ), the National Institutes of Health (NIH), and the National Institute of Nursing Research (NINR), typically have very stringent educational and experiential guidelines and requirements for principal investigators. Governmental grants are highly competitive and are allocated based upon the quality of the proposal and available funding. These grants are available for doctorate-prepared (PhD) nurse researchers and doctoral candidates (dissertation grants). Funding amounts vary significantly depending upon the type of grant and funding mechanism. For example, the RO-1 grant from the NIH supports research that has the potential to make a major impact on practice, is funded for 3 to 5 years, and does not have a funding limit. However, requests for more than $500,000 per year require special explanations, and it is expected that pilot research specific to the request for funding will have already been completed to ensure feasibility. In contrast, the NIH's R-21 grant is designed to support exploratory studies, is funded for 2 years, and has funding capped at $275,000.

Grants provided by professional and specialty nursing organizations are significantly smaller in monetary support, typically ranging from $2,500 to $10,000, with a few grants for $20,000 and up to $65,000. An advantage of organization grants is that the principal investigator is not required to have an earned doctorate degree, although many grants require that the principal investigator have at least a master's degree and an expert nurse researcher mentor. As with government grant funding, these grants are competitive and are distributed based upon quality of the proposal and available funding. Although not all organizational grants require membership in the professional or specialty organization offering the grant, most state that all things being equal, preference will be given to researchers who hold membership in the sponsoring organization.

Corporate funding of nursing research should not be overlooked. Many large corporations have a research program director and funds set aside for investigator-initiated and -led research projects. In most cases, there is a website with guidelines for submission and the application is online. The research application may not be easy to find, and often requires contact with the corporation spokesperson. Similar to organization research requests, a proposal (even

TABLE 3.3 External Funding Sources

FUNDING SOURCES	NUMBER	AMOUNT	DEADLINES
Professional Nursing Organizations			
Sigma Theta Tau International (STTI) and Local Chapter Awards	Varies	$3,000–$10,000	Varies
Nursing Research Society Awards: Midwest Nursing Research Society (MNRS), Southern Nursing Research Society (SNRS), Eastern Nursing Research Society (ENRS)	MNRS (4)	$2,500–$10,000	November 3
	SNRS (4)	$750–$5,000	Varies by Grant
	ENRS/ANF (1)	$5,000	May 1
Council for the Advancement of Nursing Science	1	$5,000	December 1
American Nursing Foundation Awards	Varies	$2,500–$10,000	May 1
National League for Nursing Awards	1	Varies	February 19
Specialty Nursing Organizations			
Medical Surgical Nurses Association	4	$5,000–$20,000	May 31
Oncology Nurses Society	3	$5,000–$25,000	September 15
Foundation for Neonatal Research and Education	Varies	$5,000	May 1
American Association of Critical-Care Nurses	4	$10,000–$50,000	Oct 31
American Association of Diabetes Nurse Educators/STTI	1	$6,000	October 1
American Holistic Nursing Association	1	$5,000	February 15
Association of PeriOperative Registered Nurses/STTI	1	$5,000	April 1
Association of Women's Health, Obstetric, and Neonatal Nurses (AWHONN)	3	$5,000–$10,000	December 1
Emergency Nurses Association (ENA) Foundation/STTI	1	$6,000	March 1
Emergence Medicine Foundation/ENA Foundation	1	$50,000	February 6
Wound, Ostomy, and Continence Nurses Society	1	Varies	February 9
Government Organizations			
National Institutes of Health (NIH)/National Institute of Nursing Research (NINR)	Varies	Varies	Varies by grant
Agency for Healthcare Research and Quality (AHRQ)	Varies	Varies	Varies by grant

if brief) must be submitted with a budget. Often, the wait period is prolonged as the corporation may need to wait until a new budget period is initiated to release funds. Corporate sponsors generally want a clinical trial agreement completed between the hospital organization and themselves. Legal services should be contacted to complete the process and careful review is needed to ensure that publication of findings remains in the control of the principal investigator and research team. The corporate team should be able to review disseminated materials (abstracts, posters, oral presentation slides, and papers submitted to peer-reviewed journals) and give advice on suggested changes, but investigators have final decision-making authority. The second area of concern of investigator-initiated and -led corporate funded studies is ensuring that the clinical trial agreement does not include language that removes the right of the hospital investigators to retain ownership of intellectual property that emerges due to the research. Corporate sponsors should own intellectual property that they brought into the research study or that they share in confidence with hospital organization investigators during the clinical trial agreement period; however, they should not be able to take ownership of hospital nurse communication shared in confidence during the clinical trial agreement period. (See the section "Legal Services" for more information.)

Presentation Funding and Support

Funding to support the presentation of findings at regional, national, and international conferences is needed as a way to encourage dissemination and to provide incentives to nurses to pursue additional studies. In general, costs associated with national presentations include airfare ($500), accommodations ($500 for 2 nights—the night before and day of the presentation), food ($75/day times 2 days), and conference registration ($350–$700). Thus the typical cost to support one nurse presenting at one conference is approximately $1,500 to $2,000. If the nursing research program expects to have five studies completed each year, it would be important to budget an additional $7,500 to $10,000 for travel/presentation support.

STATISTICAL SOFTWARE

To facilitate in-house data analysis by nurse researchers, the budget needs to include funding for software (Table 3.4). There are numerous programs available. The SPSS, although costly to purchase and maintain, is the most user-friendly program, the easiest to learn, and combines a database within the data analysis program. However, there are other programs available and the most important consideration for analysis software purchases is that nurse researchers are knowledgeable about and familiar with the uses of the purchased resources.

TABLE 3.4 Data Analysis Software

PRODUCT AND USERS	COST	COMMENTS
SPSS IBM Product *Users*: Nurses, social scientists	Varies by package: three packages include 12 month support. Price based on number of users: **Standard:** $2,530–$14,000 **Professional:** $5,000–$14,000 **Premium:** $7,500–$19,000 **Grad Pack:** Starting at $69 for the basic version Can be installed on up to two computers for a 12-month license	• Easy to learn but expensive • Standard version can handle most sophisticated and univariate and multivariate tests. However, non-linear equation modeling and SEM require the other packages • Output is well labeled and easy to interpret • Code book can be printed from database • Online learning videos and other resources
SAS SAS Institute Product *Users*: Business, government, statisticians	Multiple products: $9,000 per user for 1-year subscription; includes technical support	• Steep learning curve and expensive • Programming language is considered to be out of date and it requires ability to write some code • Very powerful system capable of most of the more complex statistical tests • Can handle extremely large datasets
Stata Stata Corp Product *Users*: Science students	Two product levels with a perpetual and a 1-year license option **Stata/IC:** $600–$1,200 **Stata/SE:** $900–$1,700	• Moderate learning curve but reasonably priced • Differences in packages are related to the number of variables and the size of the dataset. However, the IC package is fine for most studies • Free tutorials and web support available
R R Foundation Product *Users*: Finance, statisticians	Free	• Steep learning curve for a nonstatistician • Open-source program with frequent updates

A NURSING RESEARCH WEBSITE

No matter how many resources are available or how well funded a nursing research program is, the key to moving from a program that provides services to nurses who want to conduct research to a program that actually produces, disseminates, and translates research knowledge is the ability of nurses to find and use available resources. The easiest way to quickly disseminate information about the many research opportunities available within an organization is to develop an easy-to-find and access, well-organized, well-maintained intranet website.

The website should provide a variety of information and one-click links to helpful resources. Content should be organized in a logical and user-friendly manner. Information sections should include general information about the program and resources, conducting research, dissemination, required and recommended education, and research policies. Chapter 2 discusses a research intranet site as a foundational element of a sustainable nursing research program and Figure 3.1 provides the home screen of the Cleveland Clinic Nursing Research Center. A website resource requires a website programmer who can update the site as needed.

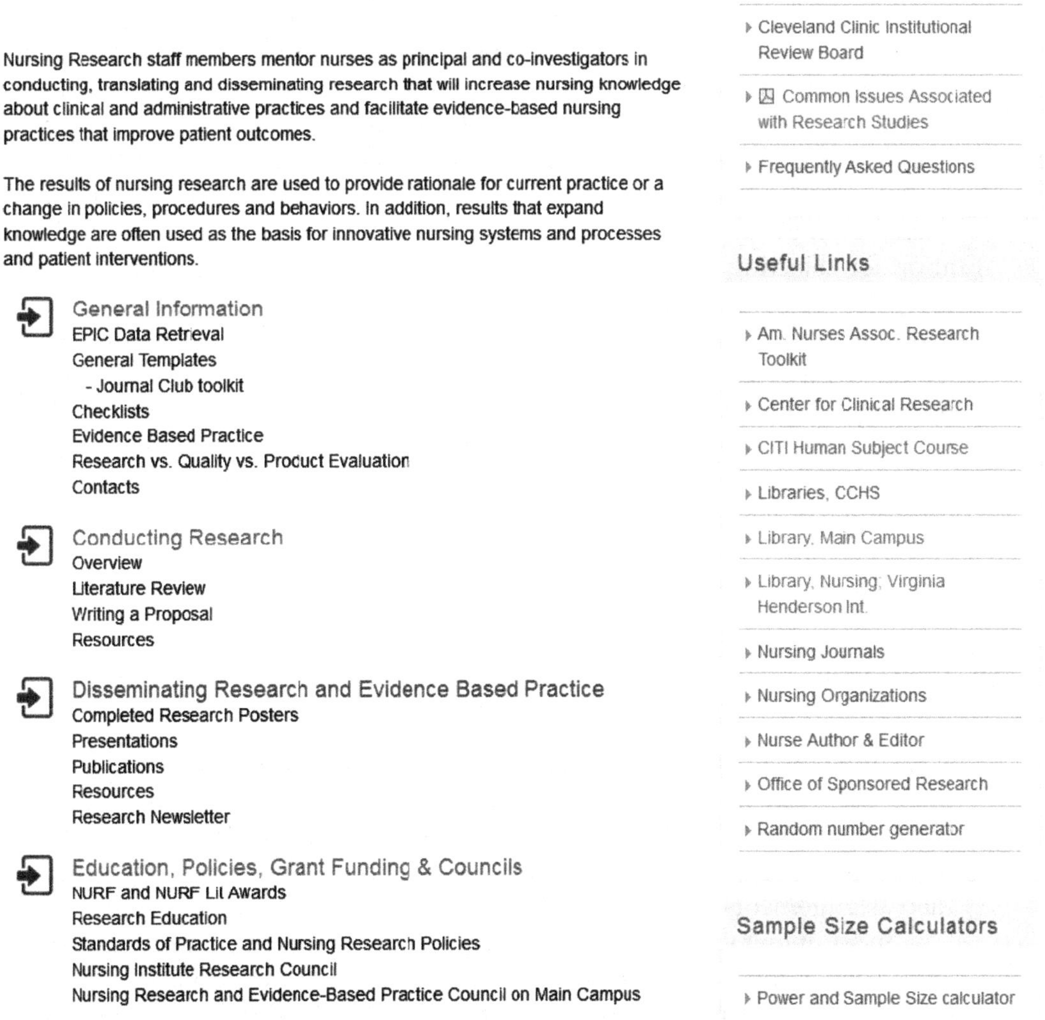

Nursing Research staff members mentor nurses as principal and co-investigators in conducting, translating and disseminating research that will increase nursing knowledge about clinical and administrative practices and facilitate evidence-based nursing practices that improve patient outcomes.

The results of nursing research are used to provide rationale for current practice or a change in policies, procedures and behaviors. In addition, results that expand knowledge are often used as the basis for innovative nursing systems and processes and patient interventions.

General Information
EPIC Data Retreval
General Templates
 - Journal Club toolkit
Checklists
Evidence Based Practice
Research vs. Quality vs. Product Evaluation
Contacts

Conducting Research
Overview
Literature Review
Writing a Proposal
Resources

Disseminating Research and Evidence Based Practice
Completed Research Posters
Presentations
Publications
Resources
Research Newsletter

Education, Policies, Grant Funding & Councils
NURF and NURF Lit Awards
Research Education
Standards of Practice and Nursing Research Policies
Nursing Institute Research Council
Nursing Research and Evidence-Based Practice Council on Main Campus

▶ Cleveland Clinic Institutional Review Board

▶ ⬚ Common Issues Associated with Research Studies

▶ Frequently Asked Questions

Useful Links

▶ Am. Nurses Assoc. Research Toolkit

▶ Center for Clinical Research

▶ CITI Human Subject Course

▶ Libraries, CCHS

▶ Library, Main Campus

▶ Library, Nursing; Virginia Henderson Int.

▶ Nursing Journals

▶ Nursing Organizations

▶ Nurse Author & Editor

▶ Office of Sponsored Research

▶ Random number generator

Sample Size Calculators

▶ Power and Sample Size calculator

FIGURE 3.1 Screen of the home page of the Cleveland Clinic Nursing Research Center website.

MISCELLANEOUS RESOURCES

In addition to personnel, funding, and statistical resources, the success of a nursing research program is enhanced by availability of survey software, library services, graphic designers, artists, and legal personnel. These resources are optional since the work they provide can be reproduced by contracted services or community businesses; however, their inclusion will enhance research and dissemination capabilities of the nursing research program.

Survey Design Resources

Survey research design methodology is a relatively easy and feasible way to answer many research questions important to clinical nurses conducting research. With the advances in electronic technology in the past decade, survey research has become very sophisticated and surveys can be developed and administered online. Data are directly downloaded for analysis. A number of software programs are available for a small or modest fee (see Table 3.5). The ability to administer surveys electronically can facilitate research and decrease time and manpower required to complete studies. Special consideration for selecting appropriate survey software is related to more than the cost. The software must be easy to use and must meet the needs of the nurse researchers who coach and mentor clinical nurses. In addition, a data export feature must be included in the license agreement. Survey Monkey Gold software is probably the most well known and one of the easiest to use. It is useful for both research surveys and general quality improvement or needs assessment surveys. REDCap is an excellent program but requires a member agreement and use is restricted to health care research. Surveys conducted to evaluate quality improvement are not supported.

Library Resources

Most, but not all, hospitals have access to some library resources. Larger hospitals may have libraries that rival many universities. A librarian and library are assets that will facilitate research by making the literature review phase quicker and easier. If library resources are not accessible within the hospital, then arrangements might be made with a local university.

In addition to organizational library resources, searches can be completed online using PubMed or Google Scholar. PubMed is a free service maintained by the National Center for Biotechnology Information located at the NIH. It includes over 20 million citations in life sciences, behavioral sciences, and other health care-related publications. Many full-text articles are available on

TABLE 3.5 Survey Software Options

PRODUCT AND RECOMMENDED OPTION	COST	COMMENTS (PROS AND CONS)
Fluid Surveys Fluidware Product *Recommend*: Enterprise	**Trial:** Free trial allows unlimited surveys but restricts number of questions to 15 and number of responses to 150 **Pro:** $215 annually. Includes most things needed for electronic survey research **Ultra:** $600 annually. Includes additional options such as phone support and more choices for questions format **Enterprise:** Price based upon number of users. This option includes the ability to download to SPSS for analysis	• Price is high for the Enterprise edition • For development and distribution of online surveys • Easy to learn with a moderate learning curve and some training information available • Only the Enterprise version includes the ability to export data to SPSS for analysis
Question Pro Question Pro Product *Recommend*: Professional	**Trial:** Free. Allows unlimited use but restricts surveys to 100 responses **Professional:** $150 annually single user **Corporate:** $900 annually single user	• Price is low for Professional edition • Can be used for online, offline, mobile, tablet, kiosk, or even scanned paper surveys • Easy to learn with a moderate learning curve and some training information available • Professional version allows export to Excel but not SPSS • Corporate version includes the ability to export to and interface with SPSS
The Survey System Aspera product *Recommend*: Professional	**Evaluation Edition** **Single user:** $49 annually **Professional Edition** **Single user:** $1,000 annually **Enterprise Edition** **Multiple users:** $2,000 annually	• Evaluation edition has limitations and can be previewed for free • Can be used for online, offline, mobile, tablet, kiosk, or even scanned paper surveys • Price is moderate to high for Professional edition • Steep learning curve and lacks an in-program training system • Can import surveys developed in MS Word
Survey Monkey *Recommend*: Gold	**Trial:** Free trial with limited number of questions and limited number of responses **Survey Monkey Gold** **Single user:** $540 annually	• Moderate price for premium features • Easy to learn and use • Appropriate for beginners and advanced survey researchers • Many free useful training services available to users • Useful for online survey delivery format and can be downloaded for paper-and-pencil survey delivery • Data export to SPSS is easy and included in the Gold edition

(continued)

TABLE 3.5 Survey Software Options (*continued*)

PRODUCT AND RECOMMENDED OPTION	COST	COMMENTS (PROS AND CONS)
REDCap Vanderbilt *Recommend*: Not applicable	**Free** for consortium members Member–users must provide the personnel to manage the system The REDCap Consortium is composed of 1,324 active institutional partners in 88 countries.	• Moderate learning curve • REDCap license is required and intended to provide access and use of the REDCap software to not-for-profit (including governmental and military) institutions and non-commercial entities and organizations who aid in the advancement of clinical and translational health care research only • No software support or training available from the software developer; however, online training is available • Supports survey development and administration as well as data entry from observation studies • Can be accessed by computer or most electronic tablets • Easy export to SPSS

this site. Google Scholar is another free search engine service that covers a wider range of scholarly publications, including but not limited to health care literature. The library may also have resources on its website that aid clinical nurses in research; for example, the ability to retrieve dissertations and other literature not available on bookshelves, multiple search engines for various disciplines and resources related to evidence-based practices. Figure 3.2 provides a screen of the Cleveland Clinic library evidence-based practice resources that were created for nurses by a librarian and the hospital organization nursing research council. It includes two short how-to videos, multiple links to sites that discuss how to review evidence for strength and quality, and various evidence-based practice models, including three models created by the nursing research program team at the Cleveland Clinic on strength of evidence, quality of evidence, and five steps to quickly rate evidence.

Graphic Design and Artist Resources

A nice to have but not necessary resource is graphic design experts and artists who develop posters for dissemination of research findings at professional conferences, artwork for journal papers and books, slide figures and tables, and newsletters or other formal print materials, such a conference syllabus or brochure. A poster is a relatively easy way to share research findings; however, they are not that easy to prepare and printing costs must be considered,

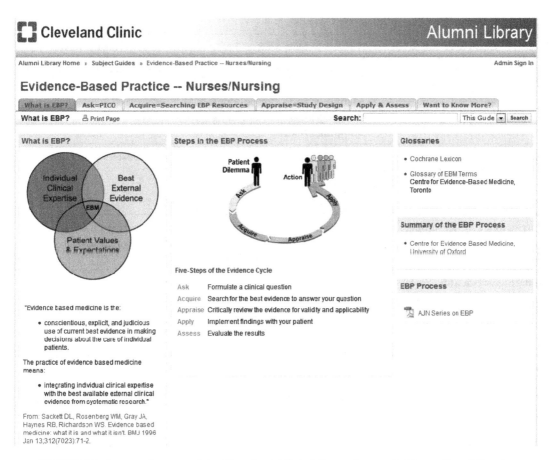

FIGURE 3.2 Screen of a page of the Cleveland Clinic Library System Evidence-Based Practice
Information. Note the themes of the six tabs.

especially when printed on cloth, rather than paper (see Chapter 9 for more information). Many poster templates can be found online (see Table 3.6 for poster resources available on the Internet). Posters can be printed at most office supply stores for a modest fee. A 3 × 6 foot nonlaminated paper color poster will cost approximately $75 to have printed; if printed on cloth, add approximately $10 per linear foot (and additional $60 for a 3 × 6 foot poster). In larger facilities that have graphic design or artist personnel, costs associated with printing posters and labor used in designing posters is often part of the services provided.

Legal Services

Legal services are not needed for all studies; however, there are multiple situations when legal representation by the hospital organization is necessary. First, as discussed earlier under funding, legal representatives should review

TABLE 3.6 Poster Template and Printing Options

COMPANY	SERVICES	WEBSITE LINK
PosterPresentations.com	• Many free templates • You do the work • Many size and color options • Both paper and cloth printing • Shipping is extra	www.posterpresentations.com
Mega Print Inc.	• Many free templates • Several size and color options • Both paper and cloth printing • Shipping is extra	www.postersession.com
Purrington, C.B., Designing Conference Posters	• Free template • Interesting "how to" section • Tips for designing your poster	colinpurrington.com/tips/poster-design
Make Signs: Scientific Posters	• Free templates • Many size and color options • Paper and cloth printing • Tips and tutorials available online • Shipping is extra	www.makesigns.com/SciPosters_Home.aspx?gclid=CJ_Fr_LQ_cMCFZGIaQod51MAiA
Genigraphics	• Free templates • Many size and color options • Paper and cloth printing • Tips and tutorials available online • Shipping is extra	www.genigraphics.com/templates

and sign off on all clinical trial agreements associated with private (for-profit) corporate-sponsored grants, whether investigator initiated and led or corporation led. In the clinical trial agreement, both parties agree to the funding amount and timeline developed for payment, freedom of nurse investigators to publish results freely, protection of intellectual property, and expectations related to confidentiality of communication shared during the course of research. In addition, hospital legal representatives should develop confidentiality disclosure agreements between the hospital organization and corporations considering funding research. Thus, before a trial agreement is initiated, a confidentiality disclosure agreement should be completed by both parties to ensure that both parties retain their intellectual property during discussions that lead to research. Second, legal representation is needed when identifiable data leave the hospital organization without explicit patient signoff. For example, nurses may initiate survey research after approval by the IRB with an allowance for verbal informed consent. Nurses may desire to transfer raw data with even one identifier to a college for assistance in analysis if the research was part of a college degree. Even if patients received verbal communication that data would leave the hospital organization, legal representatives will work

TABLE 3.7 Checklist of Hospital Organization Nursing Research Resources

RESOURCES	STRENGTH	NEED	COMMENTS
Objective and visible organizational leadership support			
Financial support (separate budget)			
• One FTE doctorate-prepared nurse researcher with experience in nursing research per ~1625 nurses			
• One FTE dedicated department director			
• One FTE administrative assistant			
• Internal funding for a minimal number of research studies annually			
• Travel budget for external presentations			
Physical space			
• Private offices with locked doors			
Equipment and supplies			
• Computers			
• Statistical analysis software			
• Locked file cabinets			
• Printer			
• Office supplies			
Organizational resources			
• Library and/or librarian*			
• Website programmer to update intranet site*			
• Biostatistician resources*			
• Sponsored research grant management system/personnel support*			
• Graphic artists*			
• Legal representation support*			

*Represents resources that are shared, not dedicated specifically to the nursing research program.

FTE, full-time equivalent.

with the receiving entity to ensure protection of human subject data. Generally, a data use agreement is completed. Third, legal services may be initiated when corporate equipment is used (borrowed) in the conduct of research.

CONCLUSION

Putting together a nursing research program requires some preparation, and it should be developed in stages, beginning with an assessment of the organization's available resources (funding, space, computers and software, library resources, and graphic design resources). It is important that foundational resources are in place before or shortly after hiring personnel; see Table 3.7 for a checklist of nursing research program resources. Careful planning in the beginning will increase the odds for success and sustainability.

REFERENCES

Albert, N. M., & Siedlecki, S. L. (2008). Developing and implementing a nursing research team in a clinical setting. *Journal of Nursing Administration, 18*(2), 90–96.

Loke, J. C. F., Laurenson, M. C., & Wai Lee, K. (2014). Embracing a culture in conducting research requires more than nurses' enthusiasm. *Nurse Education Today, 34,* 132–137.

McLaughlin, M. K., Speroni, K. G., Kelly, K. P., Guzzetta, C. E., & Desale, S. (2013). National survey of hospital nursing research, part 1. *The Journal of Nursing Administration, 43*(1), 10–17.

Christian Burchill

4

ROLE OF RESEARCH AND EVIDENCE-BASED PRACTICE COUNCILS

Scenario 1: You have been called to the chief nursing officer's (CNO) office to talk about nursing research. You helped a professor in your master's degree program conduct a research study in your hospital organization several years ago and are listed as a co-author on the published research article. Because of your "research background," the CNO (and/or the professional practice model clinical leader) thinks you have the experience and knowledge to initiate, lead, and/or invigorate the nursing department's Nursing Research and Evidence-Based Practice Council as part of a new goal toward the American Nurses Credentialing Center's Magnet® designation.

Scenario 2: You found the nursing research classes in nursing school interesting and frequently questioned evidence that supported or did not support practice. You've been talking to some clinical colleagues at your hospital and they are interested in nursing research and evidence-based practice, just like you. You think the hospital should have a nursing research and evidence-based practice council to promote advancing nursing science and high-quality evidence-based clinical practices by clinical nurses.

Scenario 3: You recently received a doctorate of nursing practice degree that required a final project with a quality focus. Your college mandated institutional review board (IRB) oversight, so you wrote a proposal and submitted it. The IRB deemed the research plan a quality initiative and closed the application. You are excited to apply the skills and knowledge you learned in your doctoral program to your clinical work setting and are happy to accept the role of reorganizing a nursing research and evidence-based practice council that had few dedicated members, no current initiatives, and a mission that was outdated and impractical.

Even if the scenarios do not sound familiar, an organized group of nurses that meets regularly for the purpose of promoting and/or conducting evidence-based practice initiatives or clinical nursing research can be unbelievably helpful in building and nurturing a hospital-based nursing research program. Depending on the organizing structure within the nursing department, it may be called a council, task force, or committee. From this point forward in this chapter, this group is referred to as a council. Regardless of the name, the goals of the council will most likely reflect nursing leadership's goals or strategic initiatives associated with a hospital-based nursing research program, primarily, to meet the vision of clinical nursing research (see Chapter 10) and aid progress in researching outcomes related to known benefits (see Chapter 1). In some hospital organizations, the nursing research council is the only structure in place to advance nursing science; there may not be a department devoted to nursing research. When this is the case, council goals or activities may center on setting up and maintaining foundational components (see Chapter 2); organizing structure, system, and process resources important to hospital-based nursing research programs (see Chapter 3); providing guidance and resources for protection of study participants (see Chapter 5) and assurance of research quality (see Chapter 6); encouraging clinical nurses to participate in and conduct nursing research studies, despite barriers (see Chapter 7); implementing changes in practice based on results (see Chapter 8); and, disseminating research findings locally and more broadly to effect change and high-quality evidence-based practices (see Chapter 9). Nursing research councils, whether established or newly created, have some unique characteristics compared to other hospital councils that may make achieving any of the aforementioned concepts a challenge. For the nursing research council to become a highly productive group, members will need to put structures in place and garner support from key personnel.

GARNERING SUPPORT

Nursing Leadership Support

The first step in the journey of developing a nursing research council is to gather support from nursing leadership. Nursing leadership may be one nursing executive or a group of executives. Leadership may also be formal or informal clinician–leaders (individuals or groups) carrying out a professional practice model or those involved in implementing and sustaining a shared-governance model. From this point forward, formal leaders within the nursing department are labeled nursing leadership, and clinical nurses who lead and participate in research councils are called clinical nurse leaders. Once established, a council requires leadership support on many levels, including managers, directors, and executive nurse leaders. In order to garner initial and ongoing support and resources, there must be clearly defined benefits for the nursing profession, the hospital, nurses, and patients. Benefits need to be clear, concise, and practical, and should match or be coordinated with the nursing department and the hospital's mission and strategic initiatives.

Support from nursing leadership usually equates to provision of resources (Saladino & Gosselin, 2014). Resources can be diverse and involve fiscal support, materials, and operational support (see Table 4.1). Simple requests involve regular meeting space, food or meals for special events, and limited support of an administrative assistant. The most important resource is time. In today's ever-changing, budget-conscious health care environment, time away from regularly assigned clinical work impacts patient care and operating budgets. Nursing research council clinical nurse leaders will need time away from assigned caregiver work or may need approval to complete council work on nonwork days. Attendance at council meetings and time to develop and participate in council activities and programs must be valued by nursing leadership. For clinical nurses, value is reflected in receiving pay for time spent in council work. Participation should not be a volunteer activity. The resource of time also entails coordination of schedules with direct supervisors and coordination of patient or administrative needs with clinical colleagues so that clinical or managerial work needs are covered when clinical nurses are attending council meetings.

TABLE 4.1 Resources That Support a Nursing Research Council

FISCAL RESOURCES	MATERIALS AND OPERATIONAL RESOURCES
• Administrative assistant presence at meetings, to set up meetings, take and type meeting minutes, and coordinate council activities, as needed	• Meeting room
	• Conference telephone or other means of long-distance communication at meetings
• Informatics technology support to develop and maintain a website of council activities	• Use of a color copier
	• Access to inclusion in nursing leadership meetings (or minutes) that provide strategic plans, revised mission statement, and current and future goals
• Costs toward an annual nursing research conference for employees or travel money to be used to support attendance at local, regional, or national nursing research meetings	• Use of a hospital computer with Internet access
	• Access to a librarian and library services (within hospital organization or paid service)
• Costs toward purchase of food, awards, books, and other resources needed to maintain the council's presence and vitality	• Central/convenient area to store paper materials associated with council activities
• Clinical nurse leader time to plan meetings	• Nursing leader presence on the council to facilitate two-way and multidisciplinary communication so that council activities and successes are shared, gaps and barriers to success are discussed, and new initiatives can be coordinated and disseminated globally
• Time for council member attendance at meetings	
• Doctorate-prepared nurse researcher (internal or external consultant) to guide, mentor, coach, and educate council members	• Access to an ethics committee/IRB (within or external to the hospital organization)
	• Policies that allow clinical nurses to be principal investigators of research protocols

IRB, institutional review board.

Nursing leadership can show support of nursing research and council initiatives by disseminating council information to managers and frontline clinicians. One great advantage of the formal nursing leadership role of authority is that people will pay more attention to their message. In the initial phases of establishing the council, and periodically throughout the life of the council, nursing leadership needs to take on visible roles of cheerleader, advocate, formal supporter, and leader so that barriers to translating evidence-based practices into clinical policies and procedures are minimized and resources needed to facilitate the conduct of nursing research by clinicians are enhanced.

Nursing leadership should provide detailed information about hospital council reporting structures and a standard format for formal documents on the council's vision, mission, objectives, goals, agenda, and meeting minutes. Examples of nursing research council documents (from within the hospital and external to the hospital) will inspire council members when they establish their own vision, mission, objectives, and goals. Reporting structure documents will show how hospital councils are structurally interrelated and help council members differentiate the nursing research council mission and goals from other councils, thereby increasing its importance to the hospital organization and nursing department.

Clinical Nursing Support

After establishing nursing leadership support for forming a new council or becoming a leader of an existing council, the council leader needs to identify nurses who have a strong interest in nursing research and evidence-based practice (Hedges, 2006). Nursing leadership may provide names of nurses being assigned to the council or who have been on the council in the past. More likely, nursing leadership may provide guidance on qualification requirements for council membership while leaving member recruitment and formalized qualification requirements up to the designated leader and council members. The leader of the nursing research council needs to keep in mind that nurses working in the hospital's outpatient settings and members of other councils are potential research council members and a great source of referrals and ideas.

Two important factors to consider before beginning the recruitment or reorganization process are the number of council members and the skill mix of council members. Both may have an impact on group productivity. The number of council members may have been predetermined by nursing leadership or the shared governance structure; for example, one member (who volunteered or was assigned) to represent each unit or department. Some hospitals open membership to all interested nursing staff members, which may result in a group that is not representative of all nurses within the hospital. In the latter situation, the council may have trouble keeping some members engaged if the will of the majority is followed. Based on research on the ideal number of members in a group, smaller groups are generally more effective and the ideal number of members lies somewhere between five and seven (Aubé, Rousseau, & Tremblay, 2011; Salas, Sims, & Shawn Burke, 2005; Wheelan, 2009). That may sound like an argument against a large number of council members, but delegating tasks to subgroups of three to six members can be an effective and efficient way for the council to achieve its goals and still allow representation from each nursing unit or department. Councils with great diversity among their membership will take longer to develop into high-functioning groups but do have the benefit of being able to provide more creative solutions; conversely, councils composed of members who already know each other develop into high-functioning groups quite quickly but may have limited creativity due to their homogeneity (Muchiri & Ayoko, 2013; Troyer & Youngreen, 2009; Wheelan & Kaeser, 1997). Although it would be ideal for the leader to select council members based on their qualifications, interests, and diversity of thought and experience, an effective leader will understand how diversity and group size influence group productivity and will use group dynamics to the council's advantage.

There are many reasons why nurses belong to a nursing research council. Some join after a restructuring process of the shared governance council system within the hospital. Others may be personally interested in nursing research, but previously were unable to act on their interest due to lack of a forum or leader. Managers, directors, or nurse executives sometimes assign nurses as the unit or division representative to the council. Nurses who are working on graduate degrees may want to join for the synergy between college requirements for research or evidence-based practice practica and council activities. Finally, nurses with master's or doctorate degrees may be interested in joining as a way of sharing their knowledge about evidence-based practice and research, and continuing their own professional growth.

Whether establishing a new council or reinvigorating an established council, identifying nurses with an interest in nursing research and evidence-based practice who are also interested in being council members can be a real challenge. Announcements about the council (and joining the council) and about nursing research in general that are posted on a nursing department website and communicated in newsletters and e-mails will only reach nurses who are actively searching for that information. Face-to-face meetings with clinical and administrative nurses will generate more interest in council participation than any other format, since face-to-face interaction starts the relationship-building process between clinical nurse leaders and council members and is generally the preferred method of communication by employees (Ean, 2010).

No matter the method in which nurses join the council, two considerations for success are: (a) understanding that nurses might bring expectations, biases, and habits from other council or workgroup experiences that will need to be addressed as they arise; and (b) members may enter the council with great enthusiasm that will need to be harnessed and nurtured. If the council is composed of a mix of people whose attitudes run from very interested and attentive to unsure of what to expect or even disinterested, clinical nurse leaders may need to tap into the personal needs of members or of the team they are representing so that goals are achieved; excitement for the council is generated; and a cohesive, high-functioning group is created. Group success is most likely when the leader demonstrates his or her passion for nursing research, dedication to the success of the council and council members, and a personal interest in ensuring the council is inclusive and valuable for council members as well as the hospital (Hedges, 2006).

Regardless of the reason for becoming the leader of the nursing research council, the leader and council members will need to spend a considerable amount of time on internal marketing. This will help identify potential new members for a newly established council or for replacing exiting members of an existing council. Additionally, clinical nurses need to be reminded regularly of council services and activities in order to see the council's relationship to their clinical practice (Hedges, 2006). Councils that are more mature in their development and advanced in understanding the research process may need to seek out clinical content experts for input on proposed or ongoing studies in order to provide useful feedback and effective oversight. These clinical content experts may be ad hoc members or full-time council members depending on their expertise and the projects being reviewed.

Since most nurses have little, if any, exposure to the nursing research process or nurse researchers in daily practice, they may feel unprepared to serve on the council despite an interest in nursing research or evidence-based practice (Swenson-Britt & Berndt, 2013). Internal marketing of the council will also help with this problem. The council leader may have to repeatedly make the case that every nurse has the ability to learn the skills necessary for council membership. Repeated exposure to nursing research and nurse researchers may help decrease any anxiety that nurses feel when they think about research (Leão, Farah, Reis, Barros, & Mizoi, 2013; Ravert & Merrill, 2008; Smirnoff, Ramirez, Kooplimae, Gibney, & McEvoy, 2007).

There are many ways to enhance clinical nurses' desire to be involved in clinical research. Encouraging clinical nurse participation in a discussion around a research or evidence-based practice paper on a topic is one way to reach out to potential council members (Aiello-Laws, Clark, Steele-Moses, Jardine, & McGee, 2010). It is paramount to choose an article that has clinical relevance on the unit, is short in length, and has a fairly simple design and statistical analysis. The goal is to allow nurses with interest in nursing research or evidence-based practice to feel more confident in their ability to fully participate in council activities. Additionally, when a council leader uses face-to-face interaction to lead a discussion about the strength of a published paper, clinical nurses can see the passion exhibited by the leader, which may be contagious. Another way to reach out to potential council members is to offer to review a research paper that is relevant to a topic being discussed at a regular unit team meeting. An example might be to attend a staff meeting when the unit is ready to implement a practice change. The council leader can discuss evidentiary support for the practice change. In this way, clinical nurses will learn the importance of evaluating the quality of evidence and better understand how research can be translated into practice. (See Chapter 8 for more information about translating research into practice.) Other venues and methods to generate interest in nursing research council membership include implementing nursing grand rounds, attending shared governance council and nurse manager meetings, and sharing research evidence that supports a new or revised policy or procedure.

In some instances, members may be garnered from nonnursing departments. Nursing research councils may benefit from being interdisciplinary (multiprofessional), especially if the council is the only hospital organization structure in place that fosters and facilitates nursing research or nurse participation in research, translates findings into clinical practice, assesses the quality of research processes, and guides nurses in dissemination. Table 4.2

TABLE 4.2 Interdisciplinary Participants on Nursing Research Councils

DISCIPLINE	ROLES
Ethics review board member	• Relate and enforce human subjects protection policies and procedures • Educate on federal regulations and local rules • Arbitrate on issues of quality versus research, protocol deviations, unanticipated problems and adverse events
Librarian	• Educate nurses about search engines and access to research papers • Develop and pay for Internet resources for the library site • Conduct searches for research projects • Search evidence-based practice resources
Informatics technology	• Provide support for accessing electronic medical record data for individual research studies • Provide devices (smartphones and tablets) that may be used in data collection • Assist with developing online survey development • Assist with database development
Doctorate-prepared academic nurse researcher	• Educate on proposal development, sampling plans, and data analysis • Provide leadership in creating grant funding paperwork, provide mentorship, and provide a letter of support • Facilitate academic–clinical partnerships in research • Mentor council members conducting a research study • Educate council members on levels of evidence when reviewing evidence for a practice change or new practice
Other health care and hospital professionals*	• Provide input and feedback on research proposals in which they have expertise • Assist in generating multidisciplinary research project development • Provide access to resources outside of the nursing department
Hospital business administrator	• Assist with grant and financial management issues • Estimate costs for research proposals • Assist with estimating cost savings in related research
Biostatistician	• Provide education on statistical and research methods for nursing research projects • Conduct statistical analyses on research projects

*Physical therapy, occupational therapy, social work, pharmacy, pastoral care, nutrition therapy.

provides a list of professionals from other disciplines and their roles on a nursing research council. When a research council is interdisciplinary, it is important to develop policies regarding decision making. Nonnurse members may be standing members with voting privileges or may be in a consultative role without decision-making authority. Alternately, nonnurse members may have adjunct status in which they are called into meetings when an agenda item requires their expertise or support.

VOICE OF A NURSE RESEARCHER

Tammy Cupit, PhD, RN-BC
Director, Nursing Research, University of Texas Medical Branch Health System, Galveston, Texas

We continue to face challenges in maintaining members (there are currently about 68 consistent members). The nursing research that is generated (four studies in 2014 and three already completed by June 2015) are conducted by nurses who contact me through my role and not through the nursing research council. Some have indicated that the council meeting time, 1 through 2:30 p.m., is very difficult to make. Council membership is composed of clinical nurses from varying areas. We sought, and continue to seek, nurses from all major areas of practice, hoping to stimulate ideas, promote diversity, and garner broad interest. Keeping the engagement level high within the membership is an ongoing struggle. I offer educational sessions each meeting, rotating journal clubs with research education sessions. The nursing research council sponsors a quarterly Bridging the Gap Between Nursing Research and Practice session where I assist them in finding a nurse researcher or team of nurses who have completed research with me, and we do presentations with breakfast and lunch. We sponsor the Nursing Showcase of Excellence once a year during Nurses' Week, where we solicit abstracts for nursing research, quality improvement, and evidence-based practice projects.

DEVELOPING A HIGH-FUNCTIONING GROUP

Effective leadership of the research council requires an understanding of some basic elements that affect group productivity. Knowledge related to how groups develop over time and the challenges leaders and members face in promoting group development will help the leader guide council members through the phases of development with as little disruption to productivity as possible. Knowledge of members' experiences in other groups and basic knowledge and interest in nursing research create a baseline understanding that leaders can build on to promote group development that is focused, productive, engaging, and based on realistic goals and expectations.

Understanding Group Development

Groups follow patterns of development over time that are similar to human development. Many theories exist as to why these patterns exist and how to identify them (Bales, 1955; Bennis & Shepard, 1956; Bion, 1961; Tuckman, 1965; Wheelan, 1996). In general, the process usually begins with a period of member dependence on the leader to establish structures that promote feeling safe when getting to know each other and the work of the group. Early dependence on the leader is followed by a period of "flight or fight." In this period, members may distance themselves from the leader or each other (by missing meetings without explanation), or create cliques, as they seek ways to become more productive. Signs of conflict or flight need to be resolved in a constructive manner to promote a productive group dynamic. Greater levels of understanding and trust are derived from the process, and in the next stage, cliques turn to effective subgroups. Additionally, member strengths are used more effectively, and the group becomes more productive. At the highest level of group development, leadership becomes more fluid, goal attainment more rapid, and productivity reaches its peak. Unlike the process of human development, group development can move forward, slide backward, or stand still. Group productivity increases as groups go higher in the developmental phases and decreases as groups regress to lower stages of development (Wheelan, 1998; Wheelan & Tilin, 1999; Wheelan, Burchill, & Tilin, 2003).

All group activity can be broken down into one of two essential elements: group structures and group tasks (Wheelan & Williams, 2003). Both exist simultaneously but vary in amount over time. Group structures are activities that strengthen the basic building blocks of group process. Policies, procedures manuals, organizational charts, and job descriptions are examples of group structures that promote group functioning. Other group structures are less obvious. Communication structures (such as to whom and how members speak during council meetings) and social structures (such as members' status and roles within the group) are important to recognize. In the early stages of group development, much of the energy of the group is given over to developing group structure.

One of the most important structures that needs to be addressed early is the decision-making process. The most common decision-making process that groups use is majority rule, in which the will of the majority determines movement on an action. Although it is a very quick and easy method for decision making, it doesn't take into account the thoughts and feelings of those opposed.

Majority rule decisions can lead to distrust or stifle creativity within the group and hamper development. A consensus decision-making model, on the other hand, takes longer to carry out but takes into account the thoughts and feelings of every council member. Reaching consensus requires that all council members feel that they have had enough input into the process that they can support the decision going forward. Consensus is not reached by a vote but by asking each member if they can agree to move forward with the current plan for action. A consensus model for decision making demonstrates that council structures and processes involve all members' input and that all members are valuable to the group, which supports group growth and productivity (Dong, Li, Xu, & Gu, 2015; Kea & Sun, 2015).

As group structures are put in place, the focus of the council can begin to shift to group tasks. Group tasks are about how the council will achieve its goals, objectives, mission, and vision. High-functioning groups are groups in which all the structures are in place to allow the group to achieve its goals efficiently and effectively. Although meeting regularly increases a group's chances of achieving its goals and completing its mission, meeting regularly or more frequently does not guarantee productivity, nor does it guarantee that a high-functioning group will remain a high-functioning group forever. Groups develop and regress over time for a variety of reasons. One of the most important functions of the leader is to understand where in the developmental process the group exists and to provide the necessary direction to help the group develop to the next highest level and prevent it from sliding backward to the previous level. Understanding group development processes is an invaluable resource for any leader. There are many excellent books available to council leaders and members so that they can understand the balance between group structures and tasks, and their roles in the process. One example is by Sue Wheelan (2016), entitled *Creating Effective Teams: A Guide for Members and Leaders*, Fifth Edition.

Understanding Member Experiences and Interests

It is paramount that the leader knows the qualifications and interests of the group so that goals and objectives are attainable. Goals and objectives that are out of reach for the council will cause frustration within the group very quickly. Consider sending out a survey to nurses who expressed interest in joining the council. A survey that asks about members previous experiences in evidence-based practices, research, and education will provide foundational knowledge that can be used in objective and goal setting. Further, understanding member experiences in other council or committee work will impact the functioning of the council. Effective leaders will come to know member strengths and weaknesses and will use that knowledge when preparing agendas. Evelyn Swenson-Britt and Andrea Berndt developed a valid and reliable survey that measures nurses' research self-efficacy as well as their institution's support for translating research into practice. The survey can be used by council leaders to learn council members' research self-efficacy, or by council members to learn hospital organization clinical nurses' research self-efficacy, or both (Swenson-Britt & Berndt, 2013).

Understanding the Council's Tasks and Functions

One key question that the council leader needs to consider early on is what exactly can and will the council do? The answer may depend on many factors: research education and experiences of council members, hospital resources available, presence of a council budget, and frequency of council meetings. These factors will affect development of the council's mission, objectives, and goals. A council composed of experienced nurse researchers will have a somewhat different but related set of challenges compared to a council composed of clinical nurses with little, if any, exposure to research and evidence-based practice. When research experience is high among council members, there is no need for basic research and evidence-based practice education, but this is rarely the case. Even a highly experienced council will face many of the same challenges affecting an inexperienced council when it comes to reaching out to clinical nurses about research and evidence-based practice–related issues.

More commonly, clinical nurses' exposure and experience with research and evaluation of evidence to determine its strength and quality is minimal. Council tasks may include time spent in understanding research and evidence-based practice terminology, developing research-related resources, and educating nurses about the research process, rather than developing a research project. If early tasks are too complicated for a novice group to understand or maintain, they may become disheartened and leave the council or decrease productivity. Lack of productivity in the early stages of the group may lead to frustration. Thus, council tasks should advance slowly as member knowledge about research grows. Readiness for the group to develop a research study that answers important nursing research questions can grow naturally from completion of early tasks that focused on nurse knowledge and identification of resources. Table 4.3 lists nursing research council tasks based on council member knowledge, exposure and practical experiences in research processes.

One task that may be a core mission for the nursing research council is to support clinician-led research (Barrett, 2010). When council members are early in their research development, the research project process should be as simple and feasible as possible; for example, a simple question with one outcome that can be answered with univariate descriptive, correlational, or comparative statistics. The project should have a high level of support from managers and no political landmines; be low cost; use a highly prevalent study population; be of high interest to many council members; and use simple, practical data-collection techniques. Council members who are not directly

TABLE 4.3 Nursing Research Council Tasks Based on Council Member Research Background

NOVICE*	MID-LEVEL	EXPERT
• Understand the levels of "strength" and "quality" of evidence to be able to score the strength and quality of evidence of research and review papers • Develop processes to enhance nurses' understanding of high- versus low-level evidence (strength and quality) of specific nursing practices • Develop journal clubs within the hospital, specific hospital units, and/or for council members • Create an intranet site and provide content on hospital resources (if not redundant with a nursing research program intranet site) • Receive education (for council members and/or all hospital nurses) on how to develop a PICO question, steps of the research process, how to use search engines to find papers on concepts/topics of interest, how to refine study aims after the literature review, and matching the research design to the research questions • Receive education (for council members and/or all hospital nurses) on how to develop an abstract, poster, or oral presentation • Work collaboratively with nurse researchers who are developing a nursing research proposal to provide information and feedback on research methods; specifically, patient/subject inclusion and exclusions, intervention implementation and data collection • Work collaboratively with nurse researchers on translating completed research into clinical practice, when appropriate	• Individual member and group nurse-led, mentor-supported research study that uses simple methodologies; for example, qualitative designs, or observational quantitative designs that use "big data" from hospital databases or single group with descriptive or correlational analysis • Grant application for novice researchers with designated mentor support • Lead journal club review of literature with expert researcher support • Group abstract writing, writing for publication with expert researcher support • Independent review of grant applications, research awards, or research abstracts with group discussion led by expert researchers • Education in research designs, advanced statistical analysis, and complex research methods • Participation on planning committees of research education conferences and workshops	• Individual member and group nurse-led research study development, implementation, dissemination, and translation • Grant application for research funding of an individual member or group project • Nurse-led multi-professional research study • Nurse-led multisite research study • Independent review of grant applications for funding • Independent review of research abstracts for research conference acceptance • Lead individual or group education on research topics • Promote new research by hospital nurses through awareness programs and award (funding) programs • Plan education events for hospital nurses (nursing research conferences or workshops)

*Most tasks are research mentor supported or led by an expert researcher.

PICO, population, intervention, comparison, outcome.

involved in research should provide encouragement and support for research team members and request updates at council meetings. Council members may assist with data collection, data entry in an electronic database, or data quality processes. Council members may guide the research team to hospital-provided research resources. During the novice stage of a research council, members will not be able to independently review a research proposal for scientific merit, protection of human subjects, or inclusion of all proposal elements. However, a review of proposal strengths, gaps, and limitations led by an experienced nurse researcher will be a great way to learn about proposal writing. Parts of the research process that council members with little experience or education in research can address are found in Table 4.3.

Council members may want to contribute to protocol development that involves clinical nurse colleagues as subjects or patients with medical conditions that match their clinical practice. For example: *Nurses are planning a research study of patients on medical–surgical units. Clinical nurses will be asked to draw blood at prescribed times. Council members can help researchers refine the protocol so that it is feasible for nurses to assist with blood draws.* Participation in protocol development may generate support for the research project and aid in data collection, once ready for patient enrollment. Nurses who want to participate in data collection but cannot complete both normal work and research study work may be more likely to develop data collection solutions that are feasible and do not incur overtime costs. The council may wish to track research studies conducted by or involving clinical nurses. Routine reporting of research activities will promote council-developed solutions to research challenges. Experienced nurse researchers in consultant–educator roles may present ethics committee–approved studies that have not been started yet, so that council members can be educated about the merits of the project and serve as champions for the research, especially on units involved in the study. Visibility of others' research studies may spark interest in the nursing research process by clinical nurses.

The nursing research council may be asked to energize clinical nurses to participate in and conduct nursing research. As research champions, council members can promote research education and discuss the benefits of research at the unit level. Members can encourage nurse researchers to include clinical nurses as co-investigators. In that way, clinical nurses can gain experience and knowledge in a nonthreatening, nonstressful manner, as they can negotiate workload. Participation in research is a hallmark of professionalism. Council members can encourage nurses to participate as subjects in research studies by completing surveys or questionnaires when prompted. Council member actions may increase survey response rates that are historically low for nurses (Kereakoglow, Gelman, & Partridge, 2013; VanGeest & Johnson, 2011). Clinical nurses can serve to refer potential research participants to investigators. In this scenario, investigators or designees would conduct procedures to enroll patients in studies but collaborative communication between clinical nurses and research investigators may create new relationships and knowledge that may increase participant referral (Jacobson, Warner, Fleming, & Schmidt, 2008). Collaborative practices may also prompt investigators to include clinical nurses as study co-investigators. Since clinical nurses must complete research education prior to participating in research, co-investigator status might increase research knowledge and skills.

VOICE OF A NURSE RESEARCHER

Tammy Cupit, PhD, RN-BC
Director, Nursing Research, University of Texas Medical Branch Health System, Galveston, Texas

Council members encourage clinical nurses in developing research ideas and then refer interested parties to me—possibly because I am the only doctorate-prepared nurse on the council. There still remains a knowledge gap that I continue to try to fill. We do not have a dedicated nurse scholars program as some other organizations do. That is something I am considering proposing. Members encourage clinical nurses to come to the council and present their proposals, which occurs about 75% of the time. I sit on the IRB and am able to provide council members with in-depth IRB guidance. The council hasn't conducted a research study yet; we are planning to this year and have started with a literature review.

GETTING STARTED

After council members are identified, the leader needs to consider how to begin the research council meeting process, including the time, place, and agenda. It is important to schedule the initial meeting at a time when most people can physically attend. Council leaders must include the thoughts and feelings of nurses who were unable to attend the inaugural meeting in person. A conference call is the easiest way to accommodate off-shift or off-day nurses, but video chat or webinar formats can be used. Online classroom formats, postings on shared drives, online voting, and blogs are other technology-based options that promote participation. Although options are available, full participation in real time face-to-face decision-making processes promotes engagement, faster group development, and more productivity (Haines, 2014; Kauffeld & Lehmann-Willenbrock, 2012).

Establishing Structures and Processes

The first meeting of a newly formed research council is a time when members get to know each other and the purpose of the council. The first order of business is member introductions. An icebreaker exercise may relax the atmosphere and encourage communication. For example, after stating their names and nursing units, group members can provide a personal statement on something research related, share their reason for joining the council, state a research question they have formed, describe their background in research and/or in implementing evidence-based practices, or what they hope to achieve as a council member. The icebreaker helps members learn about each other and mutual interests. Members may learn that they share similar knowledge and skills as others or identify the members to go to for mentoring. The process helps clinical nurse leaders of the council learn about members' clinical expertise, background knowledge, research interest, leadership potential, and about group needs and group processes. Through icebreaker communication, leaders may learn which members are boisterous or quiet and which want to be called on to speak or start conversations spontaneously.

If the purpose has not been developed, a discussion about the council's charter (vision, mission, goals, and objectives) is a great starting point. Creating council documents is nonthreatening, and promotes discussion about why the group exists and what the group hopes to accomplish. The council leader may need to prepare ideas in advance of the first meeting to provide direction about vision and mission statements, since many nurses may be inexperienced in this area. Objectives and goals should be easier for members to develop, as clinical nurses develop patient care goals as part of usual care. Leaders will do most of the talking at first but should not dominate the process or allow one or two members to dominate the process. Leaders should call on members with open-ended questions, seek their input in discussions, and validate all viewpoints so that members feel that their voices are heard. This communication style also promotes trust in the leader and others in the group. When members express constructive disagreement or seek clarity on a topic, encouraging discussion helps group members learn that they can trust each other and the leader. Posting notes on the room wall during discussions will allow members to see that all opinions matter, allow the leader to seek clarity as refinements are made, and maintain a record for council minutes. Once developed, the vision and mission statements, and objectives and goals can be summarized and displayed at the beginning of every meeting to keep the group on track (Mathieu & Rapp, 2009). A detailed discussion of charter components may be the only agenda item for the first series of council meetings or time may be split between charter discussions and educational topics. The group's interest level in charter development and research experience will help the leader decide the best format of initial meetings.

Vision and Mission

Vision and mission are often confused. The vision statement describes the overarching goal or aim for the council's work. It should be a simple, concise sentence or two that conveys the aspirations or optimal future for the work of the nursing research council. The vision statement should be broad, uplifting, and inspiring, and it should be timeless. There should not be a need to change the vision statement in the future as the council matures. A mission statement describes what the council is going to do in the present. It helps to define what makes this council different from other councils within the hospital, since it provides the purpose and objectives. A mission statement should be one or two sentences in length, and clearly state what the council will do, the recipients of their output, and how the work will be done.

The council's vision and mission may be based upon documents from the overarching shared governance council structure or from the nursing department's professional practice model. The council leader may want to share examples from other hospital organizations to stimulate discussion. Council members might desire to write their own vision and mission statements or adapt other shared council group statements by creating specificity to nursing research council work. If the vision and mission statements were developed before the first council meeting, by shared governance or other nurse leaders, members should discuss statement wording as if they were developing statements themselves. Discussion of thoughts and feeling about the vision and mission sets the tone for nursing research processes and the work of the council, and can motivate the group. Before adopting the vision and mission statements, the leader should ensure that consensus has been reached by asking each member if they can support the document as written. There are many resources available online that can help guide the development of vision and mission statements. Figure 4.1 provides an example of a vision and mission statement from the Nursing Research and Evidence-Based Practice Council of the Cleveland Clinic Florida, an academic medical center community hospital of under 200 beds.

Objectives and Goals

Objectives and goals are action items that describe in detail the way in which the council is going to meet its mission. Objectives are usually general statements about how the council will meet its mission. Goals are usually more specifically worded, are measurable, and have a completion date. An example of a council objective might be: *Council members will guide nurses in resources that facilitate the conduct of research studies.* A council goal for a novice group related to this objective might be: *Council members will provide one lunch-and-learn session each quarter this year to educate nurses on available resources used in conducting research studies.* If council members are advanced in research knowledge and skills, a council goal might be: *Council members will provide mentoring and support to novice clinical nurse investigators (principal investigator [PI] or co-PI).* As with all

---

Cleveland Clinic (CC) Florida
Nursing Research Council Strategic Plan

Mission: The mission of the CC Florida Nursing Research Council is to promote the development of nursing research studies and provide guidance for the dissemination and implementation of results as evidence-based clinical practice.

Vision: The vision for CC Florida Nursing Research Council is to ensure that CC Florida nurses are at the forefront for conducting and promoting scholarly nursing practice.

Goals and Objectives:

1. To increase the conduct, evaluation, use, and dissemination of nursing research by nurses
2. To facilitate knowledge of nursing and general clinical research as well as evidence-based practice (EBP)
3. To provide access to research resources that may aid in research conduct, evaluation, use, and dissemination
4. To stimulate inquiry of current health care topics and assist in seeking resolution for those identified problems
5. To disseminate research and EBP findings throughout the organization
6. To translate evidence into everyday practice

FIGURE 4.1 Sample Vision, Mission, Goals, and Objectives—Cleveland Clinic Florida.

decisions within the council, coming to consensus on each objective and goal allows members to feel a sense of ownership and commitment to seeing them through to completion.

For each objective, council members should ask questions to assist in goal setting. One question could be, "Considering our current level of experience and knowledge as a group, what specifically can we do to make *X* happen?" If no one can answer the question, the objective may be too broad or complicated for the group at the current point in their group cycle and should be retained for later use. For each objective, the group should create two goals. Leaders should keep members focused on realistic, attainable goals (Figure 4.1). Once developed, council goals should be reviewed at the beginning of every meeting or placed at the top of every agenda, so members stay focused on goal attainment.

At the end of the year, council members and nursing leadership can judge the council's actions based on stated objectives and goals. Objectives and goals should be reviewed yearly and updated as needed based on the accomplishments and challenges of the previous year. When objectives and goals are not completed by the end of the year, council members should determine the rationale and decide if their plans were feasible and obtainable. Council members may develop new goals for an unmet objective or simplify a complex objective. Objectives and goals that were met during the year should be actively celebrated by the group.

Bylaws

Developing bylaws is a nonthreatening way for council members to learn more about the leader, each other, and council processes. Bylaws define the actions by which all members will be held accountable. Bylaws may be based on the hospital organization's pre-existing standards or may be developed exclusively for the council. Reviewing predeveloped bylaws or writing bylaws as part of the group process allows all council members to understand their roles and responsibilities. Bylaws may include the meeting schedule, standing agenda items, methods to submit agenda items, requirements for membership, leadership presence, and record keeping. Bylaws may also include the length of time between meeting agenda availability and the next meeting, length of time between the meeting and distribution of minutes, and communication method for meeting cancellations. There are many books and online references available on processes for managing effective meetings, such as *Robert's Rules of Order* (www.robertsrules.org).

Requirements for Membership

Regardless of why nurses choose to join a nursing research council, council membership may depend on how and why the council was started. Rules about council membership may have been established by a governing body, such as the hospital organization's nursing executive council, the professional practice model governing body, or an outside accrediting agency. If membership criteria were not established prior to the first meeting, it should be addressed very early in council development. Important questions are found in Table 4.4.

Criteria for council membership may shift, based on council needs. If very few clinical nurses responded to repeated calls for membership, it may be desirable to include nonclinical nurses and nonnurses so that council processes are maintained. A benefit of requiring that all council members have a college degree is greater exposure to research. Research knowledge by some or many members may get a council up and running more quickly. Experienced nondegree nurse members and unlicensed assistive personnel may have great research ideas, and ideas about promoting and conducting nursing research and evidence-based practice in clinical settings. Bylaws need to address membership criteria and rules. Flexibility and global inclusion requirements for education, occupation, and job roles may enhance diversity in discussions, enrich decisions, promote innovation and novel research questions, and, ultimately, advance science. When joining the council, an application ensures that future members know their roles and responsibilities as council members, that they meet basic requirements, and that their manager is aware of their application for membership and is willing to provide

TABLE 4.4 Questions to Consider Related to Nursing Research Council Membership

THEMES	QUESTIONS
Nurse Criteria—General	• Will the council be exclusively composed of registered nurses? • Will the council be exclusively bedside clinical nurses? • Can advanced practice nurses, nursing administrators, and nurse educators be members or consultants? • Can doctorate-prepared nurse researchers be members or consultants? • Can licensed practical or vocational nurses and unlicensed assistive personnel be members? • Are there nursing department criteria that affect council membership? • Length of hospital service before applying? • Length of unit service before applying • History of disciplinary action in the year before applying? • *Fully meets* rating on annual performance review in the year before applying? • Can ambulatory nurses participate or only hospital-based nurses? • Is there a limitation to the number of nurses from one work area/department (operating room, intensive care units, obstetrics, medical-surgical, and pediatrics)?

Nurse Criteria—Education Background	• Are there nursing education requirements for council membership?
	  ■ Is a bachelor's degree a minimum requirement for membership?
	    – If yes, must the bachelor's degree be in nursing?
	    – If a potential member has a diploma or associate's degree and is working toward a bachelor's degree, can he or she join?
	• If non-nurse employees in the nursing department are interested in participating, can they become members?
	• Are non-nurse members held to the same education requirements as nurses (e.g., a bachelor's degree in their field)?

Member Expectations	• Do members need to be present at meetings to vote or participate in opinions toward consensus? • Are there a minimum number of meetings per year that must be attended? • Can members send an alternate colleague if they cannot attend a meeting? • If a member changes jobs within the hospital, is membership maintained? • If membership is based on completion of tasks by assigned dates, who monitors completion? • Can nurses be members if they do not currently work in the nursing department, but are hospital organization employees? • Can nonhospital research experts be invited to be members? Or consultants?
Council Leader	• Who is the designated leader? • Is the designated leader elected, assigned, or rotated among members? • Is the designated leader a clinical nurse, an advanced practice nurse, a nursing administrator, a nurse educator, a doctorate-prepared nurse scientist, or are there no criteria based on job role? • Who replaces designated leaders when they cannot attend a meeting? • Who replaces that person should he or she leave the council permanently? How does that happen?
Nursing Leadership Representative Member	• What is the expectation of the nurse executive for the nurse leader member on the nursing research council? • What connections does the nurse leader have with stakeholders who may be involved with nursing research?

time to attend meetings. Figure 4.2 is an example of the application used by Cleveland Clinic Main Campus Nursing Research and Evidence-Based Practice Council.

VOICE OF A NURSE RESEARCHER

Karen Johnson, PhD, RN
Director, Nursing Research, Banner Health, Phoenix, Arizona

Any nurse can be a member of the nursing research committee. There are some bedside nurses on the committee, but the majority of the members are CNSs and educators. The committee is charged with creating and sustaining the culture of inquiry. They review research/evidence-based practice (EBP) proposals for scientific merit and feasibility, identify mentors for projects, maintain a database of all research/EBP projects, and promote and assist with dissemination. Some of our committees use part of the agenda as a journal club.

Educating Council Members

Education about nursing research and evidence-based practice processes can be achieved many ways (Chapter 7). Many resources are available online and in nursing research books. Content can be a framework for an educational curriculum. Speakers may be hospital-based research experts or academic-based nurse researchers and biostatisticians. One method to begin the education process would be to solicit suggestions of evidence-based clinical practice problems that nurses understand. Learning about criteria used to support or refute specific practices will be of interest to clinical nurses, and may create enthusiasm to read research literature more critically. Asking council members to search through nursing policies for those that may be out of date is one way to generate clinical practice topics. Skills learned by critically reviewing the literature will be used repeatedly to review the literature as part of the process when developing a nursing research study. Skills related to searching for evidence are critical to determining if research is necessary or if current practices should be upheld. When nurses understand how findings from a review of the literature are used to prompt changes in nursing practice, they may be energized to help generate research questions as part of a council member-led research project, once ready.

Application for Membership

To be considered for Council membership, please complete and submit the following application.

Name and Credentials: (please print) _____

E-mail Address: _____ @ccf.org

Nursing Unit: _____

Tenure of Current Nursing Unit: _____

I have support for my participation in this council from my immediate supervisor.

(Required)

Name of your immediate supervisor: (please print) _____

Supervisor's Signature: _____

If selected as a member, I agree to attend meetings and actively participate in the activities of this Council to promote the generation, use, and dissemination of research at the Cleveland Clinic. I also agree to complete the CITI course within the first 6 months of membership and every 3 years. I will provide evidence of course completion to the chair or vice-chair. I understand that I will not have the benefits of membership considered for the clinical ladder program without having completed the CITI course and actively participating in the Council.

Applicant's signature: _____

FIGURE 4.2 Sample Nursing Research and Evidence-Based Practice Council Application—
       Cleveland Clinic main campus.
CITI, Collaborative Institutional Training Initiative.

Research and evidence-based practice education activities provided by the council may generate research interest among clinical nurses. Journal club activities (see Chapter 7) are common within research councils. Research and review papers are identified for hospital nursing staff to discuss each month. Council members may provide a one-page handout of paper strengths and limitations for nurses to review independently. Alternately, council members can provide a framework for conducting monthly journal clubs and allow clinical nurses on each unit to review papers independently. Another education strategy is a council-sponsored monthly lunch-and-learn session led by nurse researchers. Research topics can be selected by clinical nurses, council members, or presenters. The council can provide handouts, continuing education units, and other resources needed and work with nurse managers to increase clinical nurse participation. Nursing research newsletters produced by the council can include regular columns on clinical nurse–led research projects, evidence-based practice changes, research analysis or research methods education, translation of research findings into practice, research presentations delivered by clinical nurses at national meetings, and research awards. Finally, internal marketing of council activities can be assumed by council members. Each council member can be assigned as a liaison to one or more nursing units and attend staff and unit-based shared governance council meetings, and shift huddles to discuss nursing research and evidence-based practice initiatives and results. The number of unit contacts over the course of the year and number of attendees at meetings or huddles can be tracked and reported per year as a council outcome.

Member education and the extent to which members are prepared to promote nursing research may aid council work. As was mentioned previously, councils composed of highly experienced nurse researchers may not need basic research and evidence-based practice education. Regardless of experience level, education may include topics on (a) ethical conduct in nursing research, reading grants or proposals, reviewing abstracts, and soliciting award winners of nursing research initiatives, (b) evaluating and implementing evidence-based practices (specifically in strength and quality of research evidence), (c) writing for publication, (d) different research methods, and (e) different analysis methods (see Chapter 7). New knowledge in research allows nursing research council members to be frontline resources for clinical nurses interested in conducting research or investigating and implementing evidence-based practices.

Council Education Standards
Basic educational requirements provide council members with a common language and a basic understanding of rules, regulations, policies, procedures, and the importance of ethical treatment of human subjects who volunteer to participate in research studies. An experienced researcher, IRB member, or hospital or college ethicist can lead this discussion on a yearly basis to keep members up to date on concepts. Online human subjects protection programs, such as the Collaborative Institutional Training Initiative (CITI) developed by the University of Miami, are available. The CITI program has multiple research modules, so that research education can be customized to hospital institution needs. The basic course covers topics such as history and ethics of human subject research; IRB regulations and review process; genetics in research; vulnerable populations; and FDA regulations that affect research. Since nurses are heavily involved in social and behavioral research, CITI modules on social and behavioral human subjects' protection themes should be considered, and content will provide new knowledge about research misconduct. Completion of mandatory human subjects protection education required by the IRB has added benefits of increasing council members' understanding of research requirements and preparing them as investigators and co-investigators so they can guide others. Whether minimum research education standards are completed through self-study, online training, or by classroom methods, members' confidence in teaching unit colleagues about evidence-based nursing practices will be enhanced. Minimal educational requirements for all research council members should be determined as part of the bylaws.

Getting to Work

Once the council foundation has been laid, council work begins. Early on, agendas for meetings might focus almost entirely on research or evidence-based practice education. An outside expert may be invited to present or council members or subgroups may provide presentations on topics of expertise. Tasks assigned to members to complete before the next meeting should be simple and easy.

One way to begin council work is to have members examine their nursing policy and procedure manual for examples of policies based on expert or consensus level evidence (the lowest quality of evidence). After selecting a policy to explore further (by consensus, to promote trust and cohesion within the group), the next steps involve seeking out and evaluating evidence from available research literature. Agenda items for future meetings might include presentations by a medical librarian on how to conduct a literature search on the policy topic, a discussion on evaluating levels of evidence, or a critique of a research paper related to the policy. In this way, the group begins to learn about evaluating evidence for practice and the research process simultaneously. The group may also enjoy breaking down each section of a research paper (for congruence between sections) as part of discussion. An early focus on education rather than developing a research project will allow novice council members to learn skills to conduct, evaluate, and promote nursing research.

VOICE OF A NURSE RESEARCHER

Connie White-Williams, PhD, RN, FAAN
Director, Center for Nursing Excellence, Assistant Professor,
School of Nursing, University of Alabama at Birmingham Hospital,
Birmingham, Alabama

The purpose of our Evidence Based Nursing Practice and Research Committee is to serve as a resource for nurses interested in evidence-based practice and research and to provide opportunities that promote evidence-based nursing practice and research at University Hospital. We have a robust council mostly comprised of staff nurses. Attending at least three council meetings is a requirement of the clinical ladder program. The council meeting is held at lunch time and, up until a year ago, we offered lunch. However, economic cutbacks now prohibit this benefit. The council is sponsored by the Center for Nursing Excellence and run by a DNP-educated nurse. Engagement strategies include Evidence-Based Nursing Practice and Research Day, Manuscript Mania Days, workshops, and reward and recognition for completed projects.

SPECIAL CONSIDERATIONS IN NURSING RESEARCH COUNCILS

Nursing research councils may face some unique challenges compared to other hospital councils. Nurse researcher and council leader characteristics may affect council productivity and development. Based on job role and job category, nurse researchers and, possibly, the council leader may have higher education, experience, and position within the organization. Groups with great disparity in member status are less productive and take longer to develop compared to groups in which disparities between member status is fairly low (Wheelan, 1996; Wheelan & Johnston, 1996; Wheelan & Kaeser, 1997).

Nurse Researchers

Some nursing research councils have experienced nurse researchers in attendance at meetings. They may be hospital employees within or external to the nursing department, or they may be affiliated with a local academic institution. The group must decide on nurse researcher roles and responsibilities. Since nurse researchers have a greater understanding of and confidence in discussing the nursing research process, there may be a perception that they have higher status within the group and the group may defer to their expertise (Wheelan, 1996). The leader must make sure that clinical nurses do not acquiesce to the will of nurse researchers or seek their approval before making a decision. When nurse researchers are available to the council, their role at council meetings should be limited to consultant and educator to allow clinical nurses to lead meetings. Roles and responsibilities of nurse researchers at council meetings should be clearly defined in the bylaws so that the council does not become dominated by or dependent on the nurse researcher.

Council Leadership

The role of council leader should be delineated in the bylaws. Criteria for leader status should match the vision, mission, objectives, and goals of the council. Whenever possible, the leader should be interested in a chance to lead the group (volunteer). Additional requirements are current membership and evidence of council engagement by attending meetings, offering suggestions, and leading discussions. The council bylaws may specify the number of months or years on the council before advancing to a designated leader status or have requirements based on education, research experience, or clinical/professional ladder status. Council members may nominate people to lead the council and use a ballot to vote on the leader.

Succession planning may be enhanced by having a past leader, current leader, and a leader-elect serving simultaneously. Important information can be shared among council leaders, easing the transition from leader to leader and increasing the likelihood that the group will achieve its objectives and goals. The past leader serves as a guide for the current council leader, and the current leader mentors the leader-elect. Since the current leader sets the agenda for the council, uses his or her status to garner support from others, and holds council members responsible for assigned roles and responsibilities, the person who takes on the leader role must be comfortable having crucial conversations with council members or nursing leadership when necessary. Specific bylaw criteria should include member and leader responsibilities so that all council members and nursing leadership understand expectations.

In certain instances, the council may use a nursing leader to shepherd them through initial development. The first year or two of the council may be a difficult time, especially if there is not an adjunct nursing research program in place with resources (see Chapters 2 and 3). An experienced nursing leader can guide the council, and his or her status as a nursing leader brings understanding of hospital organization resources, comfort in communicating with nurse executives and confidence in leading a meeting (Marshall et al., 2014). As the newly formed council matures, the nursing leader needs to identify a possible council member to mentor or suggest that council members select one or more leader-elects, so that council members can gain skills in council leadership before becoming council leaders. When the nursing leader and proposed council clinical leaders feel the time is right, transition of the council leadership role should occur through voting, when possible.

Some hospitals assign a nursing leader to serve in the role of council co-chair for every council or committee as a standard practice. An assumption is often made that leadership can be shared between a clinical nurse leader and a member of nursing leadership. Shared leadership is more difficult since ultimate responsibility must rest with one person who holds accountability for actions of the council. High-functioning groups have one easily identified designated leader (Wheelan & Johnston, 1996; Wheelan & Kaeser, 1997). Perhaps a better title for a nursing leader who serves a role on the council would be that of liaison. The liaison role would entail serving as mentor to the clinical nurse leader and internal and external stakeholders, and being a keeper of records and history for the council. Although leadership cannot be easily shared, nursing leaders can demonstrate commitment to the council and their role by accepting tasks and completing them in a timely and efficient manner. Further, they can groom potential future leaders from within the organization.

When a nursing leader is assigned to the council, his or her role in decision making should be established in the bylaws. Is the nursing leader's input considered in consensus building? In a voting situation, can he or she serve to break a tie? If the designated clinical nurse leader cannot attend a meeting, do the council run the meeting according to the agenda put forth by the leader? Does the leader-elect or a council member serve as leader for that meeting, and the nursing leader provide mentorship during the meeting? Clarity on the roles, responsibilities, and expectations of leaders within the council will promote higher group functioning and productivity.

When doctorate-prepared nurse researchers are considered nurse leaders, they may complicate the council's development if they use their leader status to their favor or allow council members to acquiesce to their suggestions without debate. Regardless of a formal or informal nurse leader role on the council, member input and decision making are important; otherwise, council members may lose trust in the group process and feel that their input is not valued.

CONCLUSION

Building a nursing research and evidence-based practice council can be challenging since nurses are often novices in research processes. Once developed, a research council offers many rewards for nurses, patients, and the nursing profession in regard to increased patient safety, quality of care and outcomes, nurse professionalism, and advancement of the foundation of nursing science. Attracting and maintaining council member engagement is driven by a council leader who demonstrates passion for nursing research and evidence-based practice and is able to make research relevant in day-to-day experiences. Understanding group development processes will help the leader shepherd members toward becoming a high-functioning group with realistic objectives and goals. When council members understand their roles and responsibilities and have received core education, they can create interest and energy for nurse-led research studies. With time, council members will be able to ensure that clinical nurse colleagues on units are educated about research and evidence-based practices, have research resources available to them, and understand the importance of translating new high quality research knowledge into clinical practices.

VOICES OF NURSE RESEARCHERS

Karen L. Rice, DNS, APRN, ACNS-BC, ANP
Director, The Center for Nursing Research, Ochsner Health System, New Orleans, Louisiana

Shelley S. Thibeau, PhD, RN-NIC
Senior RN Researcher, The Center for Nursing Research, Ochsner Health System, New Orleans, Louisiana

The system nursing research council is chaired by the doctorate-prepared director of the Center for Nursing Research. The council

(continued)

VOICES OF NURSE RESEARCHERS (*continued*)

consists of a representative from each of the eight facilities within the health system (education ranges from baccalaureate to doctor of nursing practice), a senior RN researcher (doctorate-prepared) from the Center of Nursing Research, the director of the System Nursing Professional Development department (doctorate-prepared), a retired PhD scientist, a nurse IRB specialist (master's prepared), and faculty advisors from five regional nursing schools.

The addition of the nursing faculty has several advantages: it (a) bridges the gap between academic and health care system strategic priorities; (b) invites scholarly discussions regarding feasibility of student-led projects within a health care system, and (c) promotes collegiality to advance nursing science across a larger region. The role of every member on the council is to provide constructive feedback on the feasibility of nurse-initiated investigations using a feasibility checklist. Based on this feedback, the council suggests changes and/or approves the project to move forward to the IRB. The doctorate-prepared council members serve as mentors for their students as well as staff nurse–initiated projects. One challenge has been sustaining mentors for staff nurse–initiated projects. A potential strategy will be to align a doctorate-prepared nurse (Center for Nursing Research or faculty) to each facility to serve as mentor/advisor for evidence-based and/or research projects.

REFERENCES

Aiello-Laws, L. B., Clark, J., Steele-Moses, S., Jardine, S., & McGee, L. (2010). Oncology nursing society journal club how-to guide. *Oncology Nursing Society*. Retrieved from www.ons.org

Aubé, C., Rousseau, V., & Tremblay, S. (2011). Team size and quality of group experience: The more the merrier? *Group Dynamics, 15*(4), 357–375.

Bales, R. F. (1955). The equilibrium problem in small groups. In A. P. Hare, E. F. Borgatta, & R. F. Bales (Eds.), *Small Group Studies in Social Interaction*. New York, NY: Knopf.

Bennis, W. G., & Shepard, H. A. (1956). A theory of group development. *Human Relations, 9*, 415–437.

Bion, W. R. (1961). *Experiences in Groups*. New York, NY: Basic Books.

Dong, Y., Li, C., Xu, Y., & Gu, X. (2015). Consensus-based group decision making under multi-granular unbalanced 2-tuple linguistic preference relations. *Group Decision and Negotiation, 24*(2), 217–242. doi:10.1007/s10726-014-9387-5

Haines, R. (2014). Group development in virtual teams: An experimental reexamination. *Computers in Human Behavior, 39*, 213–222. doi:10.1016/j.chb.2014.07.019

Hedges, C. (2006). If you build it, will they come? Generating interest in nursing research. *AACN Advanced Critical Care, 17*(2), 226–9. doi:10.1097/01256961-2006 04000-00019

Kauffeld, S., & Lehmann-Willenbrock, N. (2012). Meetings matter: Effects of team meetings on team and organizational success. *Small Group Research, 43*(2), 130–158.

Kea, B., & Sun, B. C. (2015). Consensus development for healthcare professionals. *Internal and Emergency Medicine, 10*(3), 373–83. doi:10.1007/s11739-014-1156-6

Kereakoglow, S., Gelman, R., & Partridge, A. H. (2013). Evaluating the effect of esthetically enhanced materials compared to standard materials on clinician response rates to a mailed survey. *International Journal of Social Research Methodology, 16*(4), 301–306. doi:10.1080/13645579.2012.682430

Leão, E. R., Farah, O. G., Reis, E. A. A., Barros, C. G., & Mizoi, C. S. (2013). Academic profile, beliefs, and self-efficacy in research of clinical nurses: Implications for the nursing research program in a Magnet journey hospital. *Einstein (Sao Paulo, Brazil), 11*(4), 507–13.

Marshall, D. R., Davis, P., Cupit, T., Hilt, T., Baer, J., & Bonificio, B. (2014). Achieving added value in a knowledge-intense organization: One hospital's journey. *Nurse Leader, 12*(3), 36–42.

Mathieu, J. E., & Rapp, T. L. (2009). Laying the foundation for successful team performance trajectories: The roles of team charters and performance strategies. *Journal of Applied Psychology, 94*(1), 90–103.

Muchiri, M. K., & Ayoko, O. B. (2013). Linking demographic diversity to organizational outcomes: The moderating role of transformational leadership. *Leadership and Organization Development Journal, 34*(5), 384–406.

Ravert, P., & Merrill, K. C. (2008). Hospital nursing research program: Partnership of service and academia. *Journal of Professional Nursing, 24*(1), 54–58. doi:10.1016/j.profnurs.2007.06.014

Robert, H., Honemann, D. H., & Balch, T. J. (2011). *Robert's Rules of Order Newly Revised* (11th ed.). Retrieved from http://www.rulesonline.com

Saladino, L., & Gosselin, T. (2014). Budgeting nursing time to support unit-based clinical inquiry. *Advanced Critical Care, 25*(3), 291–296.

Salas, E., Sims, D. E., & Shawn Burke, C. (2005). Is there a "big five" in teamwork? *Small Group Research, 36*(5), 555–599.

Smirnoff, M., Ramirez, M., Kooplimae, L., Gibney, M., & McEvoy, M. D. (2007). Nurses' attitudes toward nursing research at a metropolitan medical center. *Applied Nursing Research, 20*(1), 24–31. doi:10.1016/j.apnr.2005.11.003

Swenson-Britt, E., & Berndt, A. (2013). Development and psychometric testing of the nursing research self-efficacy scale (NURSES). *Journal of Nursing Measurement, 21*(1), 4–22.

Troyer, L., & Youngreen, R. (2009). Conflict and creativity in groups. *Journal of Social Issues, 65*(2), 409–427.

Tuckman, B. W. (1965). Developmental sequences in small groups. *Psychological Bulletin, 63,* 384–399.

VanGeest, J., & Johnson, T. P. (2011). Surveying nurses: Identifying strategies to improve participation. *Evaluation & the Health Professions, 34*(4), 487–511. doi: 10.1177/0163278711399572

Wheelan, S. A. (1996). Effects of gender composition and group status differences on member perceptions of group developmental patterns, effectiveness, and productivity. *Sex Roles, 34*(9–10), 665–686. doi:10.1007/BF01551501

Wheelan, S. A. (1998). Group process and productivity. *Systemic Practice and Action Research, 11*(2), 211–213.

Wheelan, S. A. (2009). Group size, group development, and group productivity. *Small Group Research, 40*(2), 247–262. doi:10.1177/1046496408328703

Wheelan, S. A., Burchill, C. N., & Tilin, F. (2003). The link between teamwork and patients' outcomes in intensive care units. *American Journal of Critical Care, 12*(6), 527–534.

Wheelan, S. A., & Johnston, F. (1996). The role of informal member leaders in a system containing formal leaders. *Small Group Research, 27*(1), 33–55. doi:10.1177/1046496496271002

Wheelan, S. A., & Kaeser, R. M. (1997). The influence of task type and designated leaders on developmental patterns in groups. *Small Group Research, 28*(1), 94–121. doi:10.1177/1046496497281004

Wheelan, S. A., & Tilin, F. (1999). The relationship between faculty group development and school productivity. *Small Group Research, 30*(1), 59–81. doi:10.1177/104649649903000104

Wheelan, S. A., & Williams, T. (2003). Mapping dynamic interaction patterns in work groups. *Small Group Research, 34*(4), 443–467. doi:10.1177/1046496403254043

Linda J. Lewicki
Peggy Beat

5

ROLES OF THE INSTITUTIONAL REVIEW BOARD AND RESEARCH COMPLIANCE EXPECTATIONS

THE ROLE OF THE INSTITUTIONAL REVIEW BOARD

Applying for institutional review board (IRB) approval should not be perceived as a burden, but rather a joint effort to ensure the protection of human subjects engaged in research. The IRB is guided in its actions by the fundamental principles of the Belmont Report (Office of the Secretary, Department of Health, Education and Welfare [DHEW], 1979) and the federal regulations: Department of Health and Human Services (DHHS) 45 CFR 462 (referred to as "The Common Rule"), and Food and Drug Administration (FDA) 21 CFR 50 and FDA 21 CFR 56. To understand these principles and regulations, it is necessary to understand the events that led to the creation of the current IRB system.

Milestones in the History of Subject Protection

Prior to 1947, there were neither well-established ethical codes nor federal regulations for the ethical conduct of research in the United States. The Nuremberg Code (Trials of War Criminals, 1946–1949), which resulted from the Nuremberg trials of Nazi physicians who conducted human experiments during World War II, created the first internationally recognized code of human research ethics. Core principles of this Code included a favorable risk–benefit analysis, informed consent, and ability to withdraw from research participation. Despite these principles, human subject violations occurred in the United States and elsewhere. A brief synopsis of major events is summarized.

In a paper published in the *New England Journal of Medicine*, Henry Beecher (1966) described 22 studies conducted by U.S. scientists and physicians where ethical violations occurred. They included the U.S. Public Health study of the natural history of untreated syphilis in Tuskegee, Alabama; the Willowbrook hepatitis studies (1950s) involving institutionalized children with mental retardation; and the Jewish Chronic Disease Hospital studies (1960s) involving immune-compromised patients, many demented. In the Willowbrook studies, children were intentionally fed solutions made from the feces of individuals with active hepatitis. Parents of these children were told their child may not be admitted to the facility unless they agreed to this experimentation. In the Jewish Chronic Disease Hospital studies, the objective was to understand how a compromised immune system responded to cancer cells. Live cancer cells were injected without consent. Despite the publication of multiple ethical violations, it was not until public attention was focused on the Tuskegee syphilis studies that action occurred.

The DHEW funded the Tuskegee syphilis study with the intent of it being a 1-year study of the natural progression of later stage syphilis in African American men. At the time of study initiation, there was no effective treatment for syphilis. This 1-year study grew into a 40-year study (1932–1972) of a vulnerable population defined by poverty and poor education, who were not consented, were denied effective treatment when penicillin became available, and underwent many medical procedures without direct benefit. In 1972, the Tuskegee study was brought to national attention by Jean Heller of the Associated Press in articles published in the *Washington Star* and *The New York Times*. The source for the articles was Peter Buxton, a Public Health Service employee. The articles led a public outcry and served as a catalyst for a congressional investigation and subsequent regulations that created IRB review. Enrolled Tuskegee subjects filed a class-action lawsuit against the U.S. government and agreed to an out-of-court settlement. In May 1997, then-President Clinton issued an official apology on behalf of the U.S. government and held a White House ceremony for participants and their families.

For brevity, other landmark studies of human subject research violations are not presented. Readers are referred to other references, such as the U.S. government human radiation experiments,1944 to 1974 (Advisory Committee on Human Radiation Experimentation, 1995), Milgram's (Milgram, 1963; Kilman, 1967) studies (1960s) of obedience to authority, the University of Pennsylvania study on gene therapy, known as the Gelsinger case (Smith & Byers, 2002), and the Henrietta Lacks story (Skloot, 2010).

The National Research Act—1974

Senator Edward Kennedy, in 1973, led a series of public congressional hearings on biomedical and social science human experimentation that resulted in passage of the National Research Act. The impact of the act was significant as it established the National Commission for the Protection of Human Subjects of Biomedical and Behavioral Research (the "Commission") and required the DHEW (now DHHS) to codify its research policies into a single regulation: Title 45, Part 46 referred to as 45 Code of Federal Regulations (CFR) 46. This code required all institutions receiving government funding for human subject research to establish an IRB to review and determine if proposed research met regulatory requirements. The foundation for the modern IRB was established with rules for IRB composition, decision making, oversight, and documentation identified. Regulations were revised in 1978 to add additional protections for vulnerable subjects: children, pregnant women, fetuses, and prisoners. Further revisions were made to define IRB responsibilities and align FDA regulations with DHEW regulations. In 1991, the final federal policy was adopted by 16 agencies of the federal government and has since been referred to as the Common Rule. Presently, revisions to the Common Rule have been proposed and are currently in the review process (October 2015). The U.S. Department of Health and Human Services published in the Federal Registry on September 8, 2015, a Notice of Proposed Rulemaking (NPRM). Proposed changes to the Common Rule are intended to strengthen federal policy on the protection of human subjects. Comments on the proposed changes are due December 7, 2015. An implementation plan has not been defined. Some of the proposed changes in the NPRM include expansion of the categories of exempt research, rules about categories of activities that can be excluded from coverage, elimination of continuing review for some minimal risk research, improved informed consent, and expansion of the definition of human subject research to include all biospecimens. Readers are referred to the DHHS for progress on these revisions. Application of the current regulations are detailed later in this chapter.

The Belmont Report

The other significant outcome from the Commission was the creation of the Belmont Report. Although only eight pages in length, it defines ethical principles and provides the analytical framework to resolve ethical issues in human subject research. The principles are: respect for persons, beneficence, and justice. Table 5.1 provides a brief description of each principle and its application. A discussion of each principle follows, with its relevance to human subjects protections.

Respect for persons. The basic premise of this principle is that individuals are recognized as autonomous beings and should be treated as such, and individuals with diminished autonomy should be afforded protections. An autonomous person is capable of self-determination and has the ability to make judgments and choices, and to take actions based on those choices. However, autonomous individuals can only self-determine if provided accurate and complete information. Their actions/decisions must be voluntary. Some individuals have diminished capacity due to age, maturity, cognitive ability, or disease. These

TABLE 5.1 The Belmont Report

PRINCIPLES	PRINCIPLE DEFINITION	APPLICATION
Respect for Persons	Recognizing the autonomy of individuals and the need for protections for people with diminished autonomy	Participation must be voluntary. Capacity to provide consent should be assessed. Additional safeguards should be provided for those without capacity, including use of a legally authorized individual. Capacity should also be re-assessed. Informed consent is secured prior to any research interventions. Additional safeguards include respect for the privacy of the subject and the confidentiality of his or her data.
Beneficence	"Do no harm" by minimizing risks and maximizing benefits	The ratio of potential benefit to individuals or science to potential risks is appropriate. The study design eliminates or minimizes risks. Conflicts of interest are eliminated or managed.
Justice	"Fairness in distribution" of risks and benefits	Participant selection is based on protocol aims and in/ exclusion criteria, not on availability, easy access, compromised state, or manipulability. Benefits from application of research findings should be available to all.

individuals should be offered additional protections to eliminate the possibility of exploitation, including use of guardians or other legally authorized individuals who understand the situation and can represent them in research situations. Another protection is possible exclusion from research studies.

Potential subjects must be approached for research participation without undue influence. The nature of voluntarism must be maintained. Not only must complete and accurate information about the research be shared, but assessment of the interpretation and understanding of that information must also occur during the consenting process. The language used during the consent discussion and in the consent document must be understandable. An individual's understanding of information should be assessed prior to obtaining signature on a consent document. Additional safeguards and protections should be offered during the consenting process for vulnerable subjects. Besides a guardian or legally authorized individual serving in the interests of the potential participant, the services of a research subject advocate may be employed. This individual, knowledgeable of the research, the studied disease, and/or research ethics can serve as an additional resource for the potential participant during the consent process, as well as throughout the conduct of the research. Another issue related to respect is the protection of the privacy of the individual and maintenance of the confidentiality of his or her data. Lastly, respect for persons implies protections from conflicts of interest of the researcher and/or the institution where the research will take place. Conflicts should be eliminated or managed.

Beneficence.   This Belmont principle translates to more than protecting individuals from harm. Beneficence obligates researchers to maximize benefits and minimize risks to participants during the conduct of research. The benefit–risk ratio of the research must be assessed and interpreted as appropriate. It is possible there may be no direct benefit to participants but rather to society or science. Risk assessment should look at more than physical risks, and consider psychological risk, financial risk, and risk to reputation or status/position. This implies the research design must be sound to bring about valid conclusions. The proposed research must be scientifically conducted in an unbiased manner; therefore, conflicts of interest must be eliminated or managed.

Justice.   Last, the principle of justice means there must be fairness in distribution of benefits and risks in research. Risks of research should be borne equally by all likely to benefit from it. Justice demands participant selection should not be based on accessibility, availability, or manipulability. Participant selection must be related to the issue being studied. Further, any products or treatments derived from the research shall be accessible to all and not limited to those in a position to afford it. Recruitment and selection are key issues related to this principle. Application and ramifications of all three Belmont principles to researchers and to the IRB review are fully discussed later in this chapter.

Federal Regulations

The DHHS and FDA regulations are available at www.hhs.gov and www.accessdata.fdr.gov, respectively, and include policy and guidance, checklists, and decision trees. A brief summary of topics addressed in the regulations are provided.

45 CFR 46
Subpart A defines when the regulations apply; defines human subject research; IRB—membership, functions and operation, review, criteria for approval, and documentation; expedited review; suspension and termination of IRB approval; requirements for informed consent; and documentation of informed consent. Subpart B addresses additional protections for pregnant women, human fetuses, and neonates involved in research. Subpart C defines the additional protections pertaining to biomedical and behavioral research involving prisoners as subjects. Subpart D presents the additional protections for children involved as research subjects.

21 CFR Part 50
These informed consent regulations apply to all clinical investigations regulated by the FDA. It provides definitions in Subpart A, informed consent requirements in Subpart B, and additional safeguards for children in clinical investigations in Subpart D.

21 CFR Part 56
These IRB regulations include the scope and definitions of IRBs; requirements for IRB review; exemptions from IRB review; registration of the IRB and membership; IRB functions and operations, records, and reports; and administrative actions for noncompliance.

Interpretation and application of these regulations are presented with ramifications for the researcher. The regulations discussed are cited in the text.

Distinguishing Research From Nonresearch Activities

When is it necessary to go to the IRB with your proposed project/study? The definitions of research, human subject research, and a clinical investigation are found in the regulations and provide guidance when determining if investigators are engaged in research and whether an IRB submission is warranted. Table 5.2 provides DHHS and FDA definitions. Note that the DHHS uses the term "research" and the FDA uses "clinical investigation."

The distinction between research and nonresearch activities may not always be clear. Keys to the distinction are the definitions and intent of the proposed activity. The term "generalizable" knowledge defines intent. The intent of

TABLE 5.2 Federal Regulations Definition of Research

REGULATIONS	DESCRIPTION
DHHS regulations (45 CFR 46.102)	Research is the systematic investigation, including research development, testing, and evaluation, designed to develop or contribute to generalizable knowledge.
	A human subject [45 CFR 46.102 (f)] means a living individual about whom an investigator conducting research obtains (1) data through intervention or interaction with the individual, or (2) identifiable private information.
FDA regulations (21 CFR 50 and 56)	Clinical investigation means any experiment that involves a test article and one or more human subjects and that either is subject to requirements for prior submission to the FDA under section 505(i) or 520(g) of the act or is not subject to requirements for prior FDA submission under these sections of the act, but the results are intended to be submitted later to, or held for inspection by, the FDA administration as part of an application for a research or marketing permit.
	In practical terms, an activity is a clinical investigation if it involves:
	Any use of a drug, other than the use of a marketed drug in the course in medical practice; any use of a medical device, other than the use of a marketed drug in the course of medical practice; or any gathering of data that will be submitted to or held for inspection by FDA in support of a marketing application.
	A human subject means an individual who is or becomes a participant in research, either as a recipient of the test article or as a control or an individual on whose specimen an investigational device is used.
	When medical device research involves in vitro diagnostics and unidentified tissue specimens, the FDA defines the unidentified tissue specimens as human subjects.

research is the creation of new knowledge. However, some IRBs apply a broad interpretation of "generalizable" to mean the publication of findings. Publications may result from nonresearch activities, such as quality assessment and improvement projects. Every IRB should have a policy that defines research, the activities requiring IRB review, and who makes the determination. Nurses should refer to their institution's IRB (or central IRB if the hospital organization does not have its own IRB) policies. Quality assessment or improvement activities are often thought to be human-subject research and are discussed.

Quality Assessment (QA) or Improvement (QI)
QA activities tend to focus on whether existing practices meet established practice standards, either internal or nationally recognized standards. QI activities focus on assessing existing practice to improve the quality of the existing practice. Both activities may involve the review of medical record information but this activity does not define it as research. The intent of QA or QI activities is on *local* application of *existing* knowledge (such as standards) to assess or improve with focus on an institution's current practice, processes, programs, systems, or management. Findings from these local applications of existing knowledge may be published but again do not fit the definition of research. The key difference is that research is intended to create new knowledge that can be widely applied or is "generalizable" to the same population outside your setting or to other populations and settings.

Some questions that, together (all four answers must be "yes"), may help distinguish QA/QI from research include:

- What is the scope? Are there existing standards (with process or outcomes data) that allow assessment of existing practice against the standard?
- What is the purpose? Is my intent to improve existing practice, processes, systems?
- What is the benefit of my activity? Will my institution's caregivers or patients potentially benefit? (This implies that results are not generalizable externally beyond local hospital organization application.)
- What is the risk of my activity? Is the risk to caregivers or patients no greater than what is involved in standard care or ordinarily expected when practice changes are implemented?

Other activities that have local application and will not generate new knowledge include utilization reviews and outcomes analyses.

Exempt Research
Research with little or no risk to subjects may qualify for exempt status when it falls in one or more of the Federal Exemption Categories under 45 CFR 46.101(b). Research involving prisoners, pregnant women, fetuses, and human in vitro fertilization are not exempt from federal regulations because they involve vulnerable subjects [Section 101(i)]. Survey research involving children

and the observation of a minor's public behavior, unless the researcher does not participate in the activities being observed, are not exempt from federal regulations [Section 401(b)]. FDA regulations do not exempt research from IRB review except in emergency circumstances [Sec 104(c)] and taste and food quality studies [Sec 104(d)]. Table 5.3 provides categories of exempt research from the CFR.

The regulations do not identify who makes the determination whether proposed research fulfills one of the exempt categories. Therefore, it is important to review your institution's IRB policy on exempt research. Generally, an IRB member or IRB administrative staff is responsible for the determination.

TABLE 5.3 Exempt Research Categories [45 CFR 46.101(b)] From IRB Oversight/Review

THEME	DESCRIPTION
Research involving normal educational practices	Research on regular and special education instructional strategies or research on the effectiveness of or the comparison among instructional techniques, curricula, or classroom management methods conducted in commonly accepted educational settings. The research cannot involve prisoners as participants and cannot be FDA-regulated. [45CFR46.101(b)(1)]
Research involving the use of educational tests	Research involving cognitive, diagnostic, aptitude, achievement tests, surveys, interviews, or observation of public behavior unless information obtained is recorded in such a manner that human subjects can be identified, directly or through identifiers linked to the subjects and any disclosure of the human subjects' responses outside the research could reasonably place subjects at risk of criminal or civil liability, financial standing, employability or reputation. No exemption is allowed when children are involved in survey or interview procedures. No exemption is allowed when children are involved in observation of public behavior unless the investigators do not participate in the activities being observed. The research cannot involve prisoners as participants and cannot be FDA-regulated. [45CFR46.101(b)(2)][46.401(b)] Not exempt under the statements above: human subjects who are elected or appointed public officials or candidates for public office or when the federal statute requires without exception that the confidentiality of personally identifiable information be maintained throughout the research and thereafter. The research cannot involve prisoners as participants and cannot be FDA-regulated. [45CFR46.101(b)(3)]
Research involving the collection or study of existing data, documents, records, pathological specimens, or diagnostic specimens	Is exempt if these sources are publicly available or if the information is recorded by the investigator in such a manner that subjects cannot be identified, directly or through identifiers linked to the subjects. The information must exist at the time the research is proposed. The research cannot involve prisoners as participants and cannot be FDA-regulated. [45CFR46.101(b)(4)]

(continued)

TABLE 5.3 Exempt Research Categories [45 CFR 46.101(b)] From IRB Oversight/Review (*continued*)

THEME	DESCRIPTION
Research and demonstration projects	Which are conducted by or subject to federal department or agency heads, and which are designed to study or evaluate or otherwise examine [45CFR46.101(b)(5)]:
	Public benefit or service programs Procedures for obtaining benefits or services under those programs Possible changes in or alternatives to those programs or procedures, or Possible changes in methods or levels of payment for benefits or services under those programs
	In addition, the research must:
	Be conducted pursuant to specific federal statutory authority Have no statutory requirements for IRB review Not involve significant physical invasions or intrusions upon the privacy interests of participants Have authorized or concurrence by the funding agency Not involve prisoners as participants Not be FDA-regulated
Taste and food quality evaluation and consumer acceptance studies	If: Wholesome foods without additives are consumed; or
	A food is consumed that contains a food ingredient at or below the level and for a use found to be safe, or agricultural chemical or environmental contaminant at or below the level found to be safe, by the FDA or approved by the Environmental Protection Agency or the Food Safety and Inspection Service of the U.S. Department of Agriculture. In addition, the research must not involve prisoners as participants. [45CFR46.101(b)(6)] [21CFR56.104(d)]
Emergency use of a test article	Provided that such emergency use is reported to the IRB within five working days. Any subsequent use of the test article is subject to IRB review. [21CFR53.104(c)]

FDA, food and drug administration; IRB, institutional review board.

If the proposed research is granted exempt designation, no further review of the research is required unless changes are made to the research proposal, including changes in data collection and human subject's protection plan that may impact risk. A re-review will be required to determine if the research still meets exempt criteria.

IRB Review

Each hospital organization with an IRB has its own policies regarding members, including nurse membership, frequency of meetings, IRB application and proposal (including amendments) requirements, and systems of communication with principal investigators. Further, IRB policies may include who can be a principal investigator (e.g., job role or education level) and other required approvals (such as a review by the director of nursing research) prior to submission to the IRB for review.

IRB Review Methods

The IRB review can be conducted by the full board at a convened meeting or through expedited review. The DHHS regulations [Section 110(b)] allow research presenting no more than minimal risk, some continuing renewal reviews, and minor changes in previously approved research to be reviewed by expedited means. The DHHS regulations [Section 102(i)] and FDA regulations define "minimal risk" as "the probability and magnitude of harm or discomfort anticipated in the research are not greater in and of themselves that those ordinarily encountered in the daily life or during performance of routine physical or psychological examinations or tests." The Office of Human Research Protections (OHRP) further interpreted minimal risk to be relative to the daily life of a normal, healthy person. Categories of research qualifying for expedited review are included in Table 5.4. An expedited reviewer has the authority to approve, require additional information, or refer the study to a full board meeting for review. An expedited reviewer cannot disapprove a study; this determination must be made at a full board meeting.

TABLE 5.4 Research Categories Qualifying for Expedited Review [45CFR46.110]

CATEGORY	DESCRIPTION
Drugs and medical devices	Research on drugs for which an investigational new drug application (IND) is not required.
	Research on medical devices where an investigational device exemption (IDE) application or an abbreviated IDE application for a nonsignificant risk (NSF) device is not required.
Blood samples	Collection of blood samples consistent with routine clinical practice to minimize pain and risk of infections by finger stick, heel stick, ear stick, venipuncture, indwelling peripheral venous catheter already in place for clinical purposes within the following limits for volume:
	From healthy, nonpregnant adults 18 years or older who weigh at least 100 pounds. For these subjects the amounts drawn may not exceed 550 mL in an 8-week period and not more than two times per week.
	From other adults, considering age, weight, and health of the subjects, the collection procedure, the amount of blood to be collected, and the frequency with which it will be collected. For these subjects, the amount drawn may not exceed:
	The lesser of 50 mL or 3 mL per kg in an 8-week period and no more than two times per week.
Biological specimens (tissues and fluids)	Prospective collection, if for research purposes by noninvasive or minimally invasive means.

(continued)

TABLE 5.4 Research Categories Qualifying for Expedited Review [45CFR46.110] (*continued*)

CATEGORY	DESCRIPTION
Data through noninvasive or minimally invasive procedures	If data collection does not require the addition of general anesthesia or sedation for research purposes and is routinely employed in clinical practice. Examples: physical sensors applied to the surface of the body; weighing or testing sensory acuity; magnetic resonance imaging, electrocardiography, electroencephalography, thermography, detection of naturally occurring radioactivity, electroretinography, ultrasound, diagnostic infrared imaging, Doppler blood flow and echocardiography; moderate exercise; allergy skin testing; procedures in adults involving a single exposure to ionizing radiation with an effective dose not exceeding 0.1mSv (the amount typically associated with a chest x-ray).
Materials (data, documents, records, or specimens)	If research involves materials (data, documents, records, or specimens) that have been collected or will be collected for purposes other than the currently proposed research project. Examples: secondary use of data collected from another research study, secondary use of clinical or educational records, use of banked specimens in biorepositories.
Data from voice, video, digital, or image recordings	Collection of data from recordings made for research purposes.
Others	Surveys, interviews, self-reports.
	Direct and indirect observations of individual and group behavior.
	Other verbal or computer-assisted interactions or assessments.
	Noninvasive physical or behavioral tasks.
	Manipulation of the subject's environment and similar methods commonly used in cognitive, behavioral, social, ethnographic, educational, health, and epidemiologic research.

IDE, investigational device exemption; IND, investigational new drug application; NSF, nonsignificant risk.

IRB Review Criteria

IRB review criteria specified in the federal regulations apply uniformly, whether by expedited means or at a convened full board meeting; refer to Table 5.5. For each criterion, elements of an IRB review are presented to guide the researcher in submitting a complete protocol and IRB application. Table 5.5 presents five non-informed consent–related criteria from the DHHS federal regulations regarding IRB approval of research.

Application of review criteria: Medical records research.   To be complete for review by the IRB, the protocol and application for medical records minimal risk research should adequately identify the study aims; significance and rationale for the study; study population, including the inclusion and exclusion criteria; study variables and data collection sheet; data analysis plan; and consent procedures, as appropriate.

TABLE 5.5 Criteria for IRB Approval of Research (Section 45CFR46.111)*

*For approval, a determination is required that *all of the following* requirements (and descriptions in right column) are satisfied:

Risks to subjects are minimized	By using procedures that are consistent with sound research design and that do not unnecessarily expose participant to risk, and whenever appropriate, by using procedures already being performed on the participant for diagnostic or treatment purpose. • Study aims, purpose are clearly defined. • There are adequate data to justify the research. • Study design is scientifically sound and will address the study hypothesis or answer the research question. • Data collected and the statistical plan are appropriate to address the study aims. • Instruments/tools/questionnaires to be used are valid. • Sample size and statistical power are adequate. • Statistical analysis is defined and appropriate to the study aim and data collected. • Data from standard care will be used as appropriate. • Research staff has the appropriate expertise to conduct the study.
Risks to subjects are reasonable	In relation to the anticipated benefits, if any, to participants, and the importance of the knowledge that may be expected to result. • Risks and benefits are identified, described, and evaluated. • Risks are minimized by the study design, inclusion/exclusion criteria, frequency of study visits, and data collected and assessments made. • The risk–benefit ratio is acceptable.
Selection of subjects is equitable	Study population is appropriate for the purposes and setting of the study. • Inclusion/exclusion criteria are appropriate. • Minorities, women, or children are not excluded. Additional safeguards are in place to protect vulnerable subjects. Recruitment strategy is appropriate. • Persons recruiting do not have undue influence, real or perceived, on potential participants. • Advertisements contain sufficient and accurate information. • Compensation is appropriate to the level of inconveniences to be endured by the participants.
Research plan, when appropriate, makes adequate provisions for monitoring the data collected	Data monitoring is completed to ensure the safety of participants. • Plan to monitor for adverse events is defined. • As determined by the level of risk, a data monitoring committee/data safety monitoring committee is in place.
Adequate provisions to protect the privacy of subjects and to maintain the confidentiality of data	Privacy of participants is protected during recruitment, consenting, and conduct of the study. Confidentiality of participants' data is protected during recruitment, consenting, and conduct of the study. • Data will be securely stored and restricted to authorized study personnel. • HIPAA requirements will be maintained.

(continued)

TABLE 5.5 Criteria for IRB Approval of Research (Section 45CFR46.111) (*continued*)

Addresses vulnerability to coercion or undue influence	• When some or all participants are likely to be vulnerable to coercion or undue influence, additional safeguards are included in the study to protect the rights and welfare of participants.

Note: For informed consent criteria, see Table 5.6.

HIPAA, Health Information Privacy and Accountability Act; IRB, institutional review board.

The risk of medical records research is that of confidentiality of the data to be collected. Therefore, data to be collected should only be the minimum needed to answer the study aim. Storage of data should be in a secure location with restricted access limited to study personnel. Paper copies of study data should be stored in a locked location. Data entered into a computer should be password protected and also limited to study personnel. Portable devices, such as laptops or jump drives, should be encrypted so data cannot be read if the portable devices are lost or stolen.

Application of review criteria: Survey research.   As with medical records research, the protocol and application for survey minimal risk research should adequately identify the study aims; significance and rationale for the study; study population, including the inclusion and exclusion criteria; study variables and instrument, questionnaire or survey, including method of instrument, questionnaire or survey distribution and return; data analysis plan; and consent procedures, as appropriate.

Although generally minimal risk, the questions asked in a survey or questionnaire may elicit unfavorable responses such as anxiety or discomfort from participants. Therefore, the research plan should include options for respondents, including the ability to not answer survey questions viewed as inappropriate or disturbing, and a contact number for the principal investigator should be provided to participants to discuss the survey. To minimize the risk to the privacy of respondents, an anonymous survey should be considered. An anonymous survey collects no identifiable information; therefore, the research team is unable to identify the respondent. Confidentiality of survey data should be protected by adequate storage and limited access to study personnel.

If the intended participants are employees, attention to recruitment methods is required. Undue influence, whether real or perceived, may be an issue when individuals in leadership or management roles recruit or distribute study surveys or questionnaires to their subordinates. Individuals should not be placed in the position to refuse their boss by declining participation in their research. Therefore, a researcher without management roles of firing ability and performance reviews should assume recruitment and survey distribution roles.

Informed Consent

Informed consent is not a signed consent form but is a continuous process of ongoing dialogue between researchers and participants. The process begins with recruitment activities where information is first shared with potential research participants, continues with complete presentation of the research study and the consent document, and is ongoing during the conduct of the research to assess participants' continued voluntary agreement to continue participation. The process should be guided by the Belmont Report's principle of respect for persons (refer to previous discussion). The Common Rule also offers guidance and states that no investigator should engage an individual as a human subject unless effective informed consent of the potential participant or his or her legally authorized representative is obtained. The information should be shared in a manner understandable to participants, minimizing the possibility of coercion or undue influence and without exculpatory language, language where the subject is made to waive or appear to waive any legal rights or releases to investigators, sponsors, and institutions from liability for negligence. Further, regulations state individuals should have sufficient opportunity (time) to consider participation.

Likewise, as advertising materials begin the recruitment and consent process, they too should be written in understandable language without creating any undue influence, such as the promise of benefit. Most IRBs have a policy requiring IRB review and approval prior to use of any advertising materials.

A consent discussion begins with an assessment of the potential participant's capacity to provide voluntary informed consent and, if capacity is limited or absent, the use of a legally authorized representative (LAR) should be secured or a decision to not include the potential participant in the research should be made. State law and institutional policy will indicate who can serve in the role of an LAR.

The person conducting the consent interview should be a member of the research team who is fully knowledgeable of the research and able to present correct and complete information in a manner and language that is understandable to the prospective participant or his or her LAR.

The consent exchange must occur under circumstances that minimize the possibility of coercion or undue influence and be conducted in a private setting. The potential participant should be encouraged to ask questions, and the researcher should both answer questions and ask questions to prompt the prospective participant to think about participating. Asking open-ended questions of the potential participant will confirm understanding of the research and what is involved. Sufficient time should be provided to the potential participant when determining whether he or she wishes to voluntarily participate in the research. The timing of the consent interview in relationship to when the research procedures will occur should also be considered. IRB policy may prohibit or restrict same-day consenting for greater-than-minimal risk studies.

Consenting of Special Populations

Children as subjects, pregnant women, and neonates have additional regulations related to consenting. There are other populations that an IRB may consider vulnerable but for which no regulations are defined. This includes those with low literacy, health literacy, and numeracy levels; non-English-speaking subjects; and adults with diminished decision-making capacity or inability to make decisions. Regulations for informed consent in special populations require additional or alternative criteria.

Children as subjects (45 CFR 46, Subpart D). If a child is to be enrolled in a research study, the parent(s) or guardian must provide permission with the assent of the child when appropriate. "Assent" means a child's affirmative agreement to take part in a research study. State law defines the upper age limit to be considered a child.

The researcher conducting the consent interview should assess whether the potential child is capable of providing assent by considering the child's age, maturity, intellect, and psychological state. Children may be able to provide assent if they understand the interventions and/or procedures in the research. The permission of one or both parents (or guardian) will depend on the level of risk.

An IRB may approve use of an assent document that is brief and explains in child-understandable terms key concepts of the research, including: what the research is about, what will happen to the child during the research, and explanation of risks and potential benefits. The assent form should be limited to one page and use pictures and diagrams to convey study information.

Pregnant women and neonates (45 CFR 56, Subpart B). Pregnant women's consent is obtained when the research is (a) directed toward the pregnancy and holds the prospect of direct benefit to the pregnant woman; (b) the prospect of a direct benefit to pregnant women and fetuses exists; or (c) if there is no prospect of benefit for women or fetuses, the risk to the fetus is not greater than minimal and the purpose of the research is development of important biomedical knowledge that cannot be obtained by any other means.

If research holds out the prospect of direct benefit solely to the fetus, then consent of the pregnant woman and the father is obtained, unless the father is unable to consent because of unavailability, incompetence, or temporary incapacity, or the pregnancy resulted from rape or incest. In all research, when fetuses are the participants, the consent of the mother on behalf of the fetus is required. Generally, the consent of the father on behalf of the fetus is also required, except when the father's identity or whereabouts cannot be reasonably ascertained, the father is not reasonably available, or the pregnancy resulted from rape.

If the research involves neonates of uncertain viability, the legally effective informed consent of either parent of the neonate or if neither parent is able to consent because of unavailability, incompetence, or temporary incapacity, the legally effective informed consent of either parent's legally authorized representative is obtained.

When childbearing women are potential participants, risks to pregnancy and developing fetuses should be assessed and decisions made regarding inclusion or the requirements for pregnancy avoidance during and after the study should be made. Likewise, if the research procedures affect sperm structure and function, pregnancy avoidance will be necessary. The consent document should identify all risks with instructions regarding pregnancy avoidance. If risks to women (or embryo or fetus if the participant becomes pregnant) are currently unforeseeable, this should also be stated in the consent and with pregnancy-avoidance strategies defined.

Subjects with low literacy and numeracy.   A competent person who does not read and write well may be enrolled into a research study with modifications to the consent process. The informed consent document should be read to the potential participant with questions addressed and comprehension confirmed. The individual should "make his or her mark" on the consent document signifying that he or she comprehends, understands, and voluntarily agrees to participate. A witness should be present during the consent process and place his or her signature on the consent document confirming the consent process was thorough, without coercion or undue influence, and a voluntary decision to participate was made.

Non-English-speaking participants.   Potential participants who do not speak and/or read English may be approached to participate in research studies if provided complete and correct information about the study in the language understandable to them. It is required that the consent document is translated into a language understandable by non-English-speaking participants and that it contains content of the English version approved by the IRB. The IRB should be provided with a statement attesting to the accuracy of the consent to match the English version. An interpreter presenting the consent information to the participant must be conversant in both English and the language of the participant. A member of the research team is present for the consent discussion and works with interpreters to ensure the consent discussions are complete, confirms the participant's understanding of the research, and ensures that the potential participant voluntarily agreed to participate. Participants, interpreters, and research team members sign each consent form. The interpreter signs as a witness.

Adults with diminished capacity or who lack decision-making capacity.   As previously discussed, individuals with limited capacity to consent may be enrolled in research studies. The IRB must determine if the proposed research entails no significant risks, or if risks are involved, there must be, at least, a greater probability of direct benefit to participants than that of harm. Additional safeguards must also be provided. Safeguards include the use of an assent document, and use of a LAR to provide permission for study participation.

The Consent Document

The consent document serves as a tool to guide the consent discussion but also serves as a reference document for the participant during the conduct of the study. The Common Rule states basic and additional requirements for the informed consent document (see Table 5.6).

TABLE 5.6 Basic and Additional Elements of Informed Consent (Sec 46.116)

ELEMENTS	DESCRIPTION
Criteria for IRB approval	1. Informed consent will be sought and appropriately documented from each prospective subject or the subject's legally authorized representative to the extent required by the regulations
	2. Informed consent will be appropriately documented as defined by the regulations
Basic	1. A statement that the study involves research, explanation of the purposes of the research, the expected duration of participation, a description of the procedures to be followed, and identification of experimental procedures
	2. A description of any reasonable foreseeable risks or discomforts to the subject
	3. A description of any benefits to the subject or to others, which might reasonably be expected from the research
	4. A disclosure of appropriate alternative procedures or courses of treatment, if any, including their important potential risks and benefits
	5. A statement describing the extent, if any, to which confidentiality of records identifying the subject will be maintained
	6. For research involving more than minimal risk, an explanation as to whether any compensation and medical treatment are available if injury occurs, and if so, what they consist of or where further information may be obtained
	7. Identification of whom to contact for answers to questions about the research and research participants' rights including whom to contact in the event of a research-related injury to the subject
	8. A statement that participation is voluntary, refusal to participate will involve no penalty or loss of benefits to which the subject is otherwise entitled, and the subject may discontinue participation at any time without penalty or loss of benefits to which the subject is otherwise entitled

(continued)

TABLE 5.6 Basic and Additional Elements of Informed Consent (Sec 46.116) (*continued*)

ELEMENTS	DESCRIPTION
Additional elements, when appropriate	1. A statement that the particular treatment or procedure may involve risks to the subject (or to the embryo or fetus, if the participant is or may become pregnant), which are currently unforeseeable
	2. Anticipated circumstances under which the subject's participation may be terminated by the investigator without the subject's consent
	3. Any additional costs to the subject that may result from participation in the research
	4. The consequences of a subject's decision to withdraw from the research and procedures for orderly termination of participation
	5. A statement of the new findings developed during the course of the research that may relate to the subject's willingness to continue participation will be provided to the subject
	6. The approximate number of subjects involved in the study

The document must be written in lay language, and be understandable to potential participants. The IRB will stamp the consent document as approved with an expiration date. A version date, as a footer, is recommended. The version date and the IRB approval stamp assist researchers to use the current consent version. The consent document should be signed and dated by the research participant and/or the LAR, the person conducting the consent interview, and the witness, if used. A date is required to document when research activities can be initiated. Participants should be provided a copy of the consent document, and the original signed consent should be securely maintained in the research file. Some IRBs may allow the combined use of the Health Information Privacy and Accountability Act (HIPAA) Authorization elements within the informed consent document. Consult with your local IRB.

Waiver of the Requirement for Informed Consent and Waiver of the Requirement for Documentation of Informed Consent
The DHHS regulations provide the IRB with the authority to waive the requirement to obtain informed consent from subjects [Section 116(d)] and/or the requirement to have participants sign a consent document [Section 117(c)]. The IRB makes this determination by assessing risks and benefits to participants associated with the research and the consent process. The research must be minimal risk.

Other requirements that must be met for the IRB to approve a consent process that does not include, or that alters, some or all of the elements of informed consent, or waives the requirement to obtain informed consent are part of the DHHS CFRs (45 CFR 46.1116[c], 46.116[d], 46.117[c]) and FDA CFRs (21CFR 56.109[c] and 56.109[d]; Table 5.7).

TABLE 5.7 Waiver of the Requirement for Informed Consent 45 CFR 46.116(c), 46.116(d), 46.117(c) and 21 CFR 56.109(c)(1) and 56.109(d)

WAIVER CRITERIA	
The IRB must find and document the following:	The research involves no more than minimal risk to the subjects
	The waiver or alteration will not adversely affect the rights and welfare of the subjects
	The research could not practicably be carried out without the waiver or alteration
	Whenever appropriate, subjects will be provided with additional pertinent information after participation

An example where the IRB may waive the requirement to obtain informed consent is medical records research. This is minimal risk research with a risk to the confidentiality of data collected. The protocol must state how the data will be securely collected, with the minimum amount of identifiable data collected and stored, and with access limited to the research team. Additionally, data must not be shared with a third party unless totally de-identified (all protected health information [PHI]—18 HIPAA elements—are removed; see Table 6.9 for details) or a limited data set (PHI removed except for dates) is created with an executed data use agreement between the two institutions sending/receiving the data. With these protections in place, the rights and welfare of participants are protected. The volume of medical records to be reviewed and the timeframe may make it impractical to secure consent as current contact information may not be available or participants may be deceased.

An IRB may waive the requirement to have participants sign a consent document if the following conditions are met: (a) the only record linking the participant to the research is the signed consent document and the risk is potential harm from breach of confidentiality, and (b) the research involves no more than minimal risk and involves no procedure for which written informed consent is required.

Alteration to Written Consent
The same regulations already discussed allow the IRB to alter the consent process through use of an information sheet, subject letter, or phone script. This is commonly done with survey or questionnaire research.

The information sheet, subject letter, or phone script should be authored by the nurse investigator, generally someone who is familiar with the patient population. The content should mirror the basic elements of a consent document. Potential participants must be made aware they are being requested to participate in a research study with the following described: why the research is being done; why the patient is being asked to participate; what is involved in the research and how long will it take to complete the survey; risk of possible loss of confidentiality and how that risk is being minimized; statement that some questions may involve sensitive or personal information, and that they may choose not to answer all questions; statement that participation is voluntary and that the decision not to participate will have no impact on the individual's current or future care; and the name of a contact person and telephone number in case the potential subject has questions or if he or she does not wish to be contacted again.

IRB Determinations

The IRB has the authority to approve, conditionally approve pending nonsubstantive changes that can then undergo expedited review, table pending substantive changes requiring further full board meeting review, or disapprove proposed research. Tabled and conditionally approved research cannot be initiated until a response is reviewed and IRB approval is secured. Approved research will be given an approval period no more than 1 year from the date of the convened IRB meeting or expedited review. An approval of less than 1 year may be given based upon the nature of the research, degree of involved risk, and vulnerability of participants.

The IRB should be viewed as a partner to ensure the rights and welfare of research participants are protected. Contact your IRB and use it as a resource when preparing your IRB application.

VOICES OF NURSE RESEARCHERS

Connie White-Williams, PhD, RN, FAAN
Director, Center for Nursing Excellence, Assistant Professor,
School of Nursing, University of Alabama at Birmingham Hospital,
Birmingham, Alabama

An IRB representative speaks at our EBNP and Research Council meeting at least once yearly, and the IRB office offers specific hours to assist nursing staff with applications. We, in the Center for Nursing Excellence, offer workshops on how to complete an IRB application. There is a Nursing Oversight Committee in which all hospital nursing research projects are reviewed for scientific integrity and approved before submitting them to the IRB. A signed letter of approval must be submitted along with the research proposal. This approval is granted by a PhD-prepared nurse. An active research study can be audited at any time for compliance.

(continued)

VOICES OF NURSE RESEARCHERS (*continued*)

Karen L. Rice, DNS, APRN, ACNS-BC, ANP
Director, The Center for Nursing Research, Ochsner Health System,
New Orleans, Louisiana

Shelley S. Thibeau, PhD, RN-NIC
Senior RN Researcher, The Center for Nursing Research, Ochsner Health
System, New Orleans, Louisiana

The nursing research policy clearly articulates that all research
proposals that are led by a nurse or that address nursing practice
must be approved by the Nursing Research Council prior to IRB
submission. Nursing research proposals go through a review by
the Center for Nursing Research. The review process includes
(a) review by a doctorate-prepared nurse scientist and biostatistician
if indicated and (b) review and approval of the proposal and budget
by the chief nurse officer of the study site. Following the two-step
review process, the proposal is reviewed by the research council
for rigor and feasibility of adhering to study-related procedures
and completing the study. A 30-item checklist addressing six categories is used to guide protocol review, including (a) general
considerations such as: the study is congruent with strategic
imperatives, there is sufficient evidence to support the study, the
study has a sound methodology, and the principal investigator
has demonstrated competency to conduct the study; (b) financial
considerations (e.g., adequate budget to complete, sufficient
funding); (c) procedures and clinical assessment (e.g., complexity
of intervention/data collection procedures, adequate staffing);
(d) study population (e.g., defined recruitment plan, feasible sample
size); (e) case report forms/documentation requirements (e.g., electronic or paper forms, transcription, long-term document storage);
and (f) other considerations (e.g., additional space, increased nurse
burden, requires departments outside nursing).

    To ensure that all nursing research follows the approval pro-
cesses, the IRB online application system generates an authorization alert to the director of the Center for Nursing Research for all
studies submitted by a nurse as principal investigator. Without
nursing approval, the IRB application is not processed. These processes have been in place since 2006 and have been successful in
ensuring that all nursing research undergoes appropriate review
and approvals.

(*continued*)

VOICES OF NURSE RESEARCHERS (*continued*)

Mary Ann Friesen, PhD, RN, CPHQ
Nursing Research and Evidence-Based Practice Coordinator,
Inova Health System, Falls Church, Virginia

The Inova Human Research Protection Program (HRPP) sets clear expectations for research study submissions and has developed a website with multiple resources to guide novice to expert researchers. Numerous templates are available for different study designs. Nurses serve on each IRB.

RESEARCH COMPLIANCE EXPECTATIONS

Identifying and defining research is generally an easy task for experienced researchers. However, novice research nurses and even experienced nurse researchers may not be as comfortable with identifying and defining "compliance," specifically research compliance. The DHHS at 45 CFR Part 46.102(d) defines research as "a systematic investigation, including research development, testing and evaluation, designed to develop or contribute to generalizable knowledge" (Office of Human Research Protection, DHHS, 2009). Merriam-Webster defines compliance as "the act or process of complying to a desire, demand, proposal, or regimen or to coercion; conformity in fulfilling official requirements" (Merriam-Webster, 2012). Health care organizations often characterize it as formal, established program that supports their commitment to following policies and standards of conduct to ensure they are in compliance with applicable federal, state and local laws and regulations. Hence, research compliance is a meld of both concepts placed in motion.

One may wonder why a hospital organization with an IRB would need a research compliance department. Research compliance often exists as a part of the hospital's Office of Corporate Compliance. Although the Office of Corporate Compliance oversees the hospital's corporate compliance program, a research compliance team oversees the hospital's research compliance program. The compliance program guidance initiative was developed by the Office of the Inspector General (OIG) to assist the health care community in preventing and reducing fraud and abuse in federal programs (OIG DHHS, 1998). In 1991, the federal government enacted the Organizational Sentencing Guidelines, Chapter 8 of the Federal Sentencing Guidelines, in an effort to make the penalties for corporate crime both uniform and predictable (U.S. Sentencing Commission, 2013). Penalties under the Sentencing Guidelines include fines and imprisonment, as well as corporate probation, which is mandatory in the case of a business that does not have an effective compliance program in place. The Sentencing Guidelines also attempt to encourage businesses to prevent and detect criminal conduct. Each crime or violation is assigned a base fine, which is either increased or decreased based upon the presence of certain mitigating circumstances. Under the Sentencing Guidelines, an organization that has an effective compliance program may receive a substantially reduced fine, and may be able to avoid corporate probation and criminal prosecution altogether (U.S. Sentencing Commission, 2013).

In 1998, the *Federal Register* published the *Compliance Program Guidance for Hospitals* and, in 2005, a *Supplemental Compliance Program Guidance for Hospitals*. Within these compliance program guidance publications, the DHHS continues to encourage hospitals to adopt and implement a voluntary compliance program in order to significantly advance the prevention of fraud, abuse, and waste, as well as to further the fundamental mission of improving quality health care (OIG DHHS, 1998, 2005).

Likewise for research, in 2005 the DHHS published a *Draft Compliance Program Guidance for Recipients of PHS Research Awards* in the *Federal Register*. The purpose of this draft guidance was to "encourage the use of internal controls to effectively monitor adherence to applicable statutes, regulation, and program requirements" (OIG DHHS, 2005, p. 8987). Although the draft compliance program guidance report was never officially finalized, the compliance program elements are nearly identical to the compliance program guidance for hospitals, and it applies the compliance elements to the U.S. Public Health Service (PHS) research awardees. The compliance program guidance elements include (OIG DHHS, 1998, 2005):

- Development and distribution of written standards of conduct, as well as written policies and procedures that promote the hospital's commitment to compliance
- Designation of a chief compliance officer and other appropriate bodies
- Development and implementation of regular, effective education and training programs for all affected employees
- Maintenance of a process, such as a hotline, to receive complaints and adoption of procedures to protect the anonymity of complainants and to protect whistleblowers from retaliation
- Development of a system to respond to allegations of improper or illegal activities and the enforcement of appropriate disciplinary action against employees who have violated internal compliance policies, applicable statutes, regulations, or federal health care program requirements
- Use of audits and/or other evaluation techniques to monitor compliance and assist in the reduction of identified problem area
- Investigation and remediation of identified systemic problems and development of policies addressing nonemployment or retention of sanctioned individuals.

In addition, compliance program guidance for public health service award-ees included an eighth element: clear definition of roles and responsibilities within the institution's organization to ensure the effective assignment of over-sight responsibilities (OIG DHHS, 2005).

Since the compliance program guidance elements were recommenda-tions, some hospitals tailored their compliance program elements to better suit their needs and structure. The following elements and corresponding explanations provide an example of one way to personalize the compliance program guidance elements for research, keeping in mind that documenta-tion of each element is vital to providing evidence of an effective compliance program.

Risk Assessment

Risk assessment and management is the backbone of a great compliance pro-gram. Risk assessments take a lot of up-front work, but they help to ensure that compliance efforts are concentrated in the right areas. For instance, in clinical research, items to review and assess are: risk of loss of privacy or confidenti-ality; risk of protocol deviations or unreported adverse events found during inspection of drug or device studies that are regulated by the FDA; finan-cial risks associated with federally funded studies or specific requirements mandated by sponsoring federal agencies, such as the Department of Defense (DOD); risk of improper billing to Medicare if study participants are Medi-care beneficiaries; and risks of protocol compliance by high school or college students who assist with the conduct of research, due to their temporary and transient status on and off of the research, and overall knowledge base in cli-nical research.

When considering risks or exposures, it is important to consider activities on a local and national level. Local activities might include the types of research occurring within the hospital and/or researchers who conduct the research. Also important are the headline stories of exposures that occur at other organizations and risks found in a review of the DHHS OIG Work Plan for the current fiscal year. The Work Plan is typically released by the OIG each October and lists particular projects (and issues) that it hopes to address during the fiscal year. Project information related to issues cuts across departmental pro-grams, including state and local government use of federal funds; the Centers for Medicare & Medicaid Services (CMS); public health agencies; Administra-tion for Children and Families; and the Administration on Aging. For example, in 2015 the OIG began to review drug sponsors' compliance with clinical trial reporting requirements. The impetus for this project was the 2007 passing of the FDA Amendments Act (AA) (42 U.S.C. § 282(j)) that mandated registra-tion and reporting of clinical trial results in a clinical trial registry and report-ing data bank known as Clinical Trials (www.ClinicalTrials.gov). Reporting requirements via the trial registry became a resource to the FDA in assessing and monitoring drug safety and efficacy. Data reports enhance assessment of clinical trials compliance with FDA AA reporting requirements and the way that the FDA ensures that reporting requirements are met (OIG DHHS, 2015).

Monitoring and Auditing

An ongoing evaluation process is critical to a successful compliance program. Monitoring and auditing of hospital operations and activities are critical internal control mechanisms. Monitoring and auditing provide evidence of hospital compliance with applicable laws, regulations, and policies, and identify and demonstrate potential compliance issues (OIG DHHS, 1998).

There are many aspects in research that can and should be monitored or audited. For example, when research is funded by an external sponsor, expenses and payments should be monitored, much in the way that one balances a checkbook. Further, if there are research-only patient care expenses (e.g., laboratory tests that are not standard of care) or a test or procedure that are paid for by the study sponsor, monitoring of patient bills is imperative to ensure that these charges were not billed to Medicare or other third-party payers. Some examples of nonfinancial monitoring and auditing are privacy, security, and research QA (labeled QA program from here through to the end of the chapter). Hospital personnel typically conduct walk-throughs to assess privacy. For research, a bit more planning would need to occur in order to assess if study data contain identifiers, and if they do, the steps the researcher has taken to protect and safeguard patients' privacy and confidentiality. Considerations are whether data are maintained on a hospital secured network that is password protected and allows only study team members to have access and if data contain the minimal amount of identifiers, such as a medical record number or date of birth versus multiple identifiers. If data are to be shared externally with college professors and corporate study sponsors, monitoring ensures that (a) patients gave proper authorization to share data outside of the hospital, (b) data were de-identified, or (c) the IRB approved a waiver of authorization and a data use agreement was appropriately executed.

The QA program is a component of the research compliance program. The purpose of the QA program is to support departmental research programs (e.g., the nursing research program) that involve human subjects. Goals are to ensure protection of human subjects; ensure data integrity; ensure compliance with hospital policies and federal, state, and local laws and regulations, including good clinical practice guidelines; and identify education and training initiatives for investigators and clinical research staff. In addition, QA program personnel foster working relationships with principal investigators, research staff, the IRB, and research compliance.

Policies and Procedures

A code of conduct is a document that provides expectations and guiding principles for employee behavior in the workplace. A code of conduct is written and tailored toward individual hospitals and is part of the corporate compliance program. Expected behaviors surrounding research reflect a hospital commitment to ensuring integrity, compliance, and the ethical conduct of business. Thus, a hospital statement regarding research should be included in a hospital's code of conduct if research is conducted on its premises. Some code of conduct principles include legal and regulatory compliance, conflicts of interest, confidentiality, professional conduct, and responsibility (OIG DHHS, 2005). The code of conduct principles should be disseminated, read, and encouraged as part of the culture in any research program.

Imagine streets without stop signs or lights; there would be chaos and lack of order. All research programs should have policies and procedures to guide researchers in their performance of research and to help address risks. The IRB has separate human subject protection policies and procedures that generally follow federal regulations. In addition, research policies and procedures are created through the research compliance department in concert with central research offices. Before implementation, policies and procedures are reviewed by research committees and approved by the hospital's governing body, such as the medical executive committee or board of governors. Categories include human subjects themes that are not inclusive of the IRB's policies and procedures; financial management; biosafety, audits, inspections and monitoring; conflicts of interest; clinical research billing; HIPAA privacy and security; shipping of hazardous materials, electronic records including electronic signatures compliance (www.fda.gov; 21 CFR Part 11); source documentation; pharmacy; publications; and research misconduct.

It is imperative that research policies and procedures do not sit on a shelf or on an online policy and procedure management system. Policies need to be communicated to researchers, implemented when appropriate, and visible. Oftentimes, monitoring and auditing activities raise investigator awareness of research policies. Research compliance checklists can be used to evaluate researcher adherence to hospital research policies.

Program Oversight

As a part of the hospital compliance program, a compliance officer should be designated to oversee and coordinate day-to-day responsibility for the compliance program. The job role requires an appropriate level of knowledge and authority to act on particular situations and to report regularly to the hospital's governing body (OIG DHHS, 1998).

To assist the compliance officer with compliance oversight, a compliance committee may be established. Committee members should be multiprofessional and multispecialty, and include people with research administration and management skills. The compliance committee should function as an extension of the compliance officer and provide the hospital organization and individual departments with increased oversight (OIG DHHS, 1998).

In the nursing department at the Cleveland Clinic, a nursing compliance committee was developed to ensure that hospital compliance policies and procedures were followed. Further, a nursing research quality committee was formed to ensure compliance in research expectations (Chapter 6). The nursing compliance committee is led by a nursing quality leader and members include clinical leaders (associate chief nursing officers, directors, and clinical nurse specialists with multiple clinical expertise) and leaders in nursing informatics, nursing research, nursing education, and human resources. The nursing quality leader represents nursing on the hospital organization compliance committee. From a nursing research perspective, research compliance findings are reported quarterly to the hospital compliance committee, and the nursing compliance committee meets semi-annually to discuss specific nursing corporate compliance goals and issues.

Awareness, Education, and Training

Training of nurse researchers (clinical nurses who are principal research investigators), nurse or non-nurse research assistive personnel, and research administration is an important element of an effective compliance program. An education and training program ensures that employees, contractors, and other individuals function on behalf of the hospital organization, and are fully capable of executing their roles in compliance with rules, regulations, and other standards (OIG DHHS, 1998).

All researchers, research assistive personnel, and administration, when appropriate, should receive research training. General training includes privacy and security, general human subjects research, and good clinical practice. Other general training should include information that increases awareness about the research compliance program, such as the role of the compliance officer, formation of the committee, and availability of anonymous complaints mechanism (e.g., a hotline.) Specific training programs should be designed for specialized audiences. For example, personnel who manage award or contract spending should receive detailed training on grant administration, sponsored projects policies, and clinical research billing compliance. Researchers and assistive personnel who are involved with day-to-day clinical research should receive more detailed training on the protection of human subjects, IRB process, responsible conduct of research, coverage analysis, and building a study budget. Nurse-led research at the Cleveland Clinic most often involves social or behavioral concepts and factors; therefore, the social and behavioral modules of the Collaborative Institutional Training Initiative (CITI; www.CITIpro gram.org) are required before department head approval of an IRB submission. Those in charge of research can assist in identifying additional specialized areas for training. General and specific training should occur upon employment or start-up into a research role (for clinical nurses who are initiating research for the first time) and periodically, depending on learning needs. Specialized training can be individualized, on a schedule, or annually. If the hospital organization does not have an electronic education record system, research personnel or the nursing research program should maintain records of formal training completed by research personnel as part of the compliance program. Records should include attendance or completion logs, descriptions of training sessions, and copies of materials distributed at training sessions, especially if training was delivered offsite by nonhospital organization personnel. A mechanism should be established to ensure that researchers, assistive personnel, and administration receive timely training. At the Cleveland Clinic, training is reviewed yearly at annual performance reviews and is a condition of continued employment, which is consistent with federal guidelines on adherence to training requirements (OIG DHHS, 1998). Failure to comply with training requirements could result in disciplinary action.

Communication

Communication is essential for an effective compliance program. Researchers and their teams need to know whom to contact for compliance questions and issues. Typically, resolution of issues involves an escalation process. For example, when individuals identify issues, they address them with the person involved and/or communicate with their supervisor. If the issues are not resolved in the nursing department, they are generally brought to the attention of nursing research program leadership, who discuss issues with the chair and coordinator of the nursing research quality committee. In hospitals without a designated nursing research quality (compliance) committee, issues should be addressed with the hospital compliance office or officer, or submitted through a reporting hotline. The reporting hotline should have the ability for the reporter to remain anonymous, as desired. Open communication increases the hospital's ability to identify and respond to research compliance concerns (OIG DHHS, 1998).

Researchers, assistive personnel, and administration must be able to ask questions and report problems. Hospital officials, department leaders, or other supervisors must respond to employee concerns and should serve as a first line of communication. The research program should adopt open-door policies to foster dialogue between management and employees. To encourage communications, confidentiality and nonretaliation policies should be distributed to all. Open lines of communication between the compliance officer and employees are equally important to the successful implementation of a compliance program.

The OIG encourages the use of hotlines, e-mails, newsletters, suggestion boxes, and other forms of information exchange to maintain open lines of communication. In addition, an effective employee exit interview program could be designed to solicit information from departing employees regarding potential misconduct and suspected violations of the hospital's policies and procedures. Information regarding how to access the corporate compliance reporting mechanism should be posted in a central and obvious area (OIG DHHS, 1998).

Enforcement and Corrective Action

When noncompliance to research policies and procedures occurs there should be consistent application of education and/or disciplinary actions that deter future acts of noncompliance. Intentional and material noncompliance should not be tolerated; and sanctions for violations could range from verbal warnings to suspension, termination, or other sanctions, as appropriate. Each situation must be considered on a case-by-case basis, taking into account all relevant factors, to determine an appropriate response (OIG DHHS, 1998).

Violation of the research compliance program, failure to comply with applicable federal or state law, and other types of misconduct threaten the violator's, hospital's, and research program's reputations in the scientific and research community, and may lead to a suspension of research activities until an investigation is concluded. Upon receipt of reasonable indications of suspected noncompliance, it is common for research compliance personnel to assist with a prompt investigation of the allegations to determine whether there was a material violation of applicable law or of the requirements of the compliance program. As appropriate, the investigation may include an assessment of internal controls, a corrective action plan, a report and repayment to the government, and/or a referral to law enforcement authorities or regulatory bodies. If misconduct is substantiated with credible evidence and after a reasonable inquiry, and it is believed that the conduct may violate criminal, civil, or administrative law, the hospital should promptly report the misconduct to appropriate authorities within a reasonable period. In the case of research misconduct, this includes reporting to the appropriate institutional body that may include the office of research integrity.

Roles and Responsibilities in Research Awards

It is especially important that roles and responsibilities regarding use of research awards be clearly defined and understood. Defining roles and responsibilities promotes accountability and is essential to the overall internal control structure of the research program. Research programs should clearly delineate the responsibilities of all persons involved with the conduct of research, including both administration or department personnel with oversight responsibility and principal investigators and other personnel who are engaged in research. Clearly defined roles and responsibilities assist research programs in fulfilling their legal responsibility to comply with federal requirements, removing any uncertainty as to the precise responsibility of all individuals involved in the research enterprise. It can also assist individuals in defending against allegations that they recklessly disregarded federal requirements. Roles and responsibilities for each position should be clearly communicated and accessible. Inclusion of roles and responsibilities in the research program's written procedures and in its formal training and education program could accomplish this objective (OIG DHHS, 2005).

CONCLUSION

The scope of a research compliance program concentrates on issues that fall under the title of research compliance and administration, meaning those issues involving the application of laws, regulations, and other program requirements that affect several aspects of research. The term compliance can be used broadly to include human subject research, conflicts of interest, research misconduct, intellectual property issues, and sponsor terms and conditions. A serious, meaningful, and effective compliance program may require a significant commitment of time and resources from researchers, personnel, and administration in addition to research compliance. Since compliance programs focus on preventing research conduct fraud and abuse through education, monitoring, auditing, and reporting, the commitment of time is justified. Ultimately, research compliance is the responsibility of every researcher, research assistive personnel, and administrator.

An effective research compliance program addresses the government's and research community's mutual goals of ensuring good stewardship of federal funds, improving administration of grants, and demonstrating to employees and the community at large the hospital organization's commitment to honest and responsible research conduct. Research compliance goals may be achieved by identifying and correcting unlawful and unethical behavior at an early stage; encouraging employees to report potential problems and allowing for appropriate internal inquiry and corrective action; minimizing financial loss to the government and any resulting financial loss to the institution;

and, through early detection and reporting, reducing the possibility of government audits or investigations regarding unallowable payments or fraud that could have been prevented at an early stage.

Hospitals may take differing approaches to how they monitor compliance issues and comprise their compliance committee, and whether they include compliance for research misconduct and human and animal subject protections as part of a single compliance program. The compliance measures adopted by research programs should be tailored to fit the unique environment of the program (including its organizational structure, operations, and resources, as well as prior enforcement experience). In short, research programs should adapt the objectives and principles underlying the measures outlined in this chapter to their own particular circumstances. Often, research compliance is involved in every element by drafting policies and procedures, communicating changes or updates in regulations, providing education, organizing training sessions, and monitoring or auditing research studies. In some instances, if there is a risk or exposure for the entire hospital, research compliance will monitor that risk across the hospital, such as HIPAA Privacy and Security. Research compliance's role is to assist and advise in creating the program; however, there is an expectation that leaders of research programs and departments must draft a plan, tailor it to the uniqueness of the research they are conducting, prioritize program elements, and then implement the program.

REFERENCES

Advisory Committee on Human Radiation Experimentation. (1995). *Final Report*. U.S. Government Printing Office.

Beecher, H. (1966). The Ethics of Research, *New England Journal of Medicine, 274*, 1354–1360.

Compliance. (2012). In *Merriam-Webster.com*. Retrieved from: http://www.merriam-webster.com/dictionary/compliance

Department of Health, Education, and Welfare. Office of the Secretary. (1979). *The Belmont Report: Ethical Principles and Guidelines for the Protection of Human Subjects of Research*. The National Commission for the Protection of Human Subjects of Biomedical and Behavioral Research. Retrieved from http://www.hhs.gov/ohrp/humansubjects/guidance/belmont.html

Department of Health and Human Services. (1997). Code of Federal Regulations. Title 45A—DHHS and Part 46—Protection of Human Subjects.

Department of Health and Human Services. Office of Inspector General. (2015). *Work Plan. Fiscal Year 2015*. Retrieved from website: https://oig.hhs.gov/reports-and-publications/archives/workplan/2015/FY15-Work-Plan.pdf

Food and Drug Administration. (1999). *Code of Federal Regulations*. Title 21, Chapter 1—Food and Drug Administration, DHHS; Part 50—Protection of Human Subjects.

Food and Drug Administration. (1999). *Code of Federal Regulations*. Title 21, Chapter 1—Food and Drug Administration, DHHS; Part 56—Institutional Review Boards.

Kilman, H. C. (1967). Human use of human subjects: The problem of deception in social psychological experiments. *Psychological Bulletin, 67,* 1–111.

Milgram, S. (1963). Behavioral study of obedience. *Journal of Abnormal and Social Psychology, 67,* 371–8.

Office of Human Research Protections, Department of Health and Human Services. (2009, July 14). Code of Federal Regulations. Title 45 Public Welfare. Part 46 *Protection of Human Subjects*. Definitions (46.102). Retrieved from http://www.hhs .gov/ohrp/humansubjects/guidance/45cfr46.html#46.102

Office of Inspector General, Department of Health and Human Services. (1998). Publication of the OIG compliance program guidance for hospitals. *Federal Register 63*(5), 8987–8998. Retrieved from http://oig.hhs.gov/authorities/docs/cpghosp.pdf

Office of Inspector General, Department of Health and Human Services. (2005). OIG supplemental compliance program guidance for hospitals. *Federal Register 70*(19), 4858–4876. Retrieved from https://oig.hhs.gov/fraud/docs/complianceguidance/ 012705HospSupplementalGuidance.pdf

Office of Inspector General, Department of Health and Human Services. (2005). Draft OIG compliance program guidance for recipients of PHS research awards. *Federal Register 70*(227), 71312–71320. Retrieved from http://oig.hhs.gov/fraud/docs/ complianceguidance/PHS%20Research%20Awards%20Draft%20CPG.pdf

Skloot, R. (2010). *The immortal life of Henrietta Lacks*. New York, NY: Crown Publishers.

Smith, L., & Byers, J. F. (2002). Gene therapy in the post-Gelsinger era. *Journal of Nursing Administration's Health, Law, Ethics, and Regulations 4,* 104–110.

Trials of War Criminals before the Nuremberg Military Tribunals under Control Council Law No. 10, Vol 2, Nuremberg, October 1946–April 1949. Wash. DC: US G.P.O., 181–182. Retrieved (date) from www.hhs.gov/ohrp/archive/nurcode.html

U.S. Sentencing Commission. (2013). Chapter 8; Sentencing of Organizations. In *2013 U.S.S.C. Guidelines Manual* (pp. 489–532). Washington, DC: Office of Public Affairs. Retrieved from website: http://www.ussc.gov/training/organizational-guide lines/2013-ussc-guidelines-manual

Joel D. Roach

6

QUALITY OVERSIGHT OF NURSING RESEARCH

At the heart of a strong nursing research program is quality oversight of research practices and procedures. Quality oversight involves the development and application of processes and resources that support optimal conduct of research. Quality oversight can increase adherence to compliance requirements and reduce occurrence of research issues. Quality of care and patient safety are core values that affect the reputation of hospital organizations (The Office of Inspector General [OIG] of the U.S. Department of Health and Human Services [DHHS] and The American Health Lawyers Association [AHLA], 2007). Nursing research subjects are often hospital or ambulatory patients and hospital employees (especially nurses) in the hospital organization. When research processes require high accountability, research safety and quality are assured. Important elements for successful quality oversight of nursing research is discussed in this chapter.

RESEARCH QUALITY COORDINATOR ROLE

The research quality coordinator (RQC) role is integral to comprehensive nursing research quality management. The RQC is interested in improving nurse researcher knowledge about quality expectations related to standard operating procedures (SOPs), good clinical practice (GCP) guidelines, and other applicable regulatory requirements that protect the rights and welfare of study participants. During study start-up and quality monitoring visits, the RQC evaluates research activities to ensure research compliance with federal guidelines and local policies. The RQC also stresses the importance of adherence to protocols as approved by an institutional review board (IRB). When compliance recommendations are aligned with evidence-based practices and written policies and standards that reflect high-quality research, nurse principal investigators (PIs) can trust that data collected will be of high quality and most importantly, that patients will be protected from harm. The RQC can provide database optimization support to PIs to enhance the quality of data entry in preparation for analysis. Finally, the RQC can be used to educate novice PIs at research study start-up. At study start-up, the RQC can provide knowledge, offer guidance in systems and processes associated with study requirements for data collection, and enhance organization of data collection processes and materials. Thus, the RQC can provide comprehensive ancillary support to nurses that begins after study approval by the IRB and continues to data submission for study analysis. The comprehensiveness of RQC services during study start-up enables doctorate-prepared nurse researchers to allocate a greater portion of time mentoring nurses and coordinating research activities that are beyond the scope or capabilities of the RQC. The work performed by an RQC is critical to a successful nursing research program. For this reason, when the program is small and there are only a few active IRB-approved research projects, the doctorate-prepared nurse researcher must carry out RQC responsibilities as part of his or her role.

By assessing the overall quality of the program, the RQC can prioritize initiatives aimed at easing some burdens associated with research start-up and data collection. He or she can minimize protocol deviations and unanticipated problems, minimize errors that are preventable and modifiable, and create order and systematic processes related to research process steps. The RQC uses department meetings, study start-up meetings, quality monitoring visits, newsletters, documents, and e-mail to communicate quality best practices and compliance expectations to members of the nursing research program and all nursing personnel.

The RQC role is collaborative and involves coordination with many research stakeholders. Prior to meeting with the study team, the RQC will review each protocol and discuss nuances with the PI's nurse researcher mentor to

VOICE OF A NURSE RESEARCHER

Mary Ann Friesen, PhD, RN, CPHQ
Nursing Research and Evidence-Based Practice Coordinator,
Inova Health System, Falls Church, Virginia

There is an infrastructure in place at Inova to monitor compliance with required research procedures via post-approval monitoring. The Research Quality Improvement Team performs both random quality reviews of active research studies and for-cause reviews under the direction of the IRB and the human research protection program (HRPP). Quality monitoring procedures enhance the protection of research subjects.

ensure all research methods related to start-up, data collection, and electronic database work are carried out using high-quality research processes. The RQC may need to work with quality subject matter experts in the nursing research program to evaluate quality risks and develop targeted solutions to overcome identified gaps. Additionally, nurse PIs and nurse researcher mentors should seek out the RQC as needs arise. After the role is established, the RQC will be a powerful catalyst for the continuous improvement of the nursing research program.

RESEARCH STUDY START-UP COMMUNICATION

Study start-up meetings are designed to give the PI and study team individualized education to prevent quality issues from occurring. Meetings are beneficial for new investigators and investigators who completed prior research but are using different study methods in the current research. Start-up meetings are necessary whenever the research design is a randomized controlled trial, as this design can be complex and investigators often need support when preparing for subject enrollment and data collection. The PI and study team will learn how to recognize and avoid common pitfalls, and can apply quality practices that ensure they adhere to IRB requirements. Study start-up meetings reduce the risk of adverse compliance observations that could occur during routine quality-monitoring activities and external audits. In many cases, the RQC can show investigators how to develop electronic files of patients who were approached and declined participation and those who met exclusion criteria, to minimize approaching a research subject more than one time. The RQC may discuss developing a document that ensures collection of data needed for a Consolidated Standards of Reporting Trials (CONSORT) diagram (www .consort-statement.org). Aggregate information collected will be used in a published report when editors require a figure that outlines study enrollment.

A regulatory binder checklist developed specifically for a nursing research program is a practical tool that can be used to facilitate study start-up discussions. This customizable checklist contains research compliance requirements and provides references to standard operating procedures, GCP guidelines, IRB requirements, and other applicable regulations. As can be seen in Table 6.1, the sections (dividers) on the Cleveland Clinic checklist include: binder organization, IRB documentation, approved study documents, research protocol, study staff responsibilities, data storage and security, and sponsor correspondence. The first section, binder organization, covers the specific order of binder content, including titles of labels for dividers. The approved study documents section encourages PIs to file IRB approved and stamped (if applicable) case report forms (CRFs). In the approved study documents section, approved study protocols should be filed, each listed with a version number. In this way, the study team will be better able to ensure current protocol adherence and be able

TABLE 6.1 Nursing Research Regulatory Binder Checklist Criteria

1 Binder Organization

- Dividers for all sections labeled:
    1. IRB Documentation
    2. Approved Study Documents
    3. Research Protocol
    4. Study Staff Responsibilities/Training
    5. Sponsor Correspondence (if applicable)

2 IRB Documentation

- All IRB correspondence on file: signed/dated applications, responses, approvals (ICH GCP: 4.9.4, 8.2.7)

- Current letter of study approval or annual continuing renewal

- Initial IRB approval letter (ICH GCP 8.2.7)

- Is there a copy of a completed Applicant Signature Page in the file for each investigator (externally sponsored studies) and subinvestigator? 21 CFR 54.4; 21 CFR 312.64 (d)

3 Approved Study Documents

- IRB-stamped approved *current* version of the ICF

- IRB-stamped approved *current* version of the CRFs

- IRB-stamped approved *current* flyers, posters, advertisements, etc. (if applicable)

4 Most recent version of the research protocol (ICH GCP 8.2.7)

- Previous versions of the protocol (if any)

- All protocol versions, dated

5 Study staff responsibilities/training

- Delegation of authority log—list of clinical staff delegated to perform study related duties (ICH GCP: 4.1.5; 4.2.4)*

- Have each research team member sign his or her own initials (ICH GCP 8.3.24)

- Substantiation of appropriate allocation of responsibilities (e.g., licensure, certification, training)

- Documentation of the study staff training (in-services) ICH GCP: 4.1.5; 4.2.4

6 Data Storage and Security

- Handle research data in a manner that protects the privacy and confidentiality of research subjects (all staff, sponsor)

- Use minimal necessary PHI—Keep research data in a locked cabinet or storage space accessible only to study staff

- Keep electronic research files on a secure computer network drive (in harmony with policies and SOPs)

- If traveling with research data, carry CRFs in a code-locked briefcase (or similar alternative)

7 Sponsor Correspondence (if applicable)

- Confirmation that a copy of correspondence to and from the sponsor is in the study file ICH GCP: 4.9.4; 8.2.9; 8.3.4

- Documentation of financial agreement between the investigator/institution and the sponsor of the trial

CRF, case report form; GCP, good clinical practice; ICF, informed consent form; ICH, International Conference on Harmonization; IRB, institutional review board; PHI, protected health information; SOPs, standard operating procedures.

to chronicle the protocol's history of revisions after IRB approval. At the start-up meeting, the RQC will provide tips for protocol deviation prevention, such as filing amendments and receiving IRB approval before implementing a change to the protocol, and conducting all research procedures within the time frame specified in the protocol. Recommendations during the study start-up meeting should be tailored to the unique needs of each study. Table 6.2 provides study management best practices. The study staff responsibilities section is reserved for written communication, algorithms, study checklists, reminders, and other correspondence that the PI and other research team members require to promote continuity of research processes and standardization. The safe data storage and security section aims to protect the privacy and confidentiality of research subjects. The following paragraph provides specific questions that could promote or enhance data security measures. The last section, sponsor correspondence, is used to retain all written correspondence between the PI and funding sponsor that includes contracts and signatures. Correspondence through e-mail or regular mail without signatures can be saved electronically. Finally, there should be columns on the checklist for "yes," "no," and "notes," so PIs can provide any details to themselves or the team on study history.

Safe data storage and security are major study start-up considerations. The PI must evaluate environmental factors and make determinations about data storage. Is there a secure place, such as a locked cabinet, where CRFs can be stored? Will only assigned study staff have access to study data? If data need to move between sites, will it be transported in a password-secured briefcase? Have efforts been made to de-identify data or use the minimal amount of protected health information (PHI) possible? Do the computers used for data storage have a firewall, and is information stored on a secure local network (provided by the hospital organization)? The PI will want to stay within the parameters of any local policies governing data security and electronic technology use. Data security measures may be included in local nursing research program SOPs.

At the Cleveland Clinic, routine study start-up meetings were initiated in the second quarter of 2013. Figure 6.1 provides a graph of 2013 protocol deviations in relation to pre- and postimplementation of study start-up meetings. In the first quarter of 2013, one minor protocol deviation was reported, and in the second quarter, two unanticipated problems occurred. After implementing study start-up meetings, there were no self-reported or discovered protocol deviations or unanticipated problems throughout the remainder of 2013. As a quality process, study start-up meetings can bring clarity to study expectations for investigators and study teams and hold value.

Study staff training is a major start-up topic that deserves distinct attention. The PI is responsible for adequately training all study staff so that each member of the research team is qualified to perform study-related duties. In addition, PIs must maintain documentation of training in the research regulatory file. The reference to training may include a history of meeting dates, discussion topics and notes. A continuous plan for research team training and ongoing education may be necessary throughout the course of each study. In situations where

TABLE 6.2 Study Management Best Practices and GCP References

ISSUE PREVENTION CONSIDERATIONS	DETAILS AND RATIONALE	GCP REFERENCES
• All pertinent information (a history of the study) in the regulatory file	• Regulatory files, subject files, recruitment logs, informed consent documents, any document that contains PHI.	ICH GCP 4.9.4; 8.2.2; 8.3.2
• Keep an electronic or printed copy of all materials submitted to the IRB	• Keep IRB response correspondence in the regulatory files, or file electronically.	ICH GCP 8.3.3; 8.3.4
	• IRB materials that do not include signatures are maintained within an electronic (or paper) binder. Materials with signatures must be kept in a *paper-based* regulatory binder.	ICH GCP 8.2.2; 8.2.6; 8.3.24
• Submit IRB applications for annual study renewals or study close-out to the IRB 30 days before study expiration	• Submit a summary of research compliance issues that occurred over the previous year (e.g., unanticipated problems, protocol deviations, adverse events).	ICH GCP 4.10.1; 5.17.3 8.4.2
• Use your hospital organization's e-mail address to communicate study-related information to all study investigators, statisticians, and other research personnel and stakeholders	• Information in personal e-mail servers are subject to the conditions of the host server. Any e-mail that contains PHI that is sent to or from your personal e-mail address is automatically considered a breach of confidentiality.	ICH GCP 5.5.3 (d)
• Submit an amended recruitment plan to the IRB if the current plan is not working or is inadequate	• Implement the amended enrollment plan after IRB approval to prevent a protocol deviation.	ICH GCP 4.4.1; 4.5.1; 4.5..2
• Comply with all regulatory policies related to data use and retention, investigator oversight and human research source documentation; if the study is sponsored by a funding agency/ group, it must also comply with regulatory policies	• Investigators must learn study-related responsibilities, educate the research team, and oversee compliance to IRB standards.	ICH GCP 4.5.1; 4.9.7; 5.5.3 (a–g); 5.5.4
• Adhere to all applicable regulatory requirements for reporting SAEs, AEs, unanticipated problems, protocol deviations, or breach of confidentiality within the required time	• Requirements are established by the IRB/IEC policy, the protocol, local SOPs, the sponsor (when applicable), GCP guidelines, code of federal regulations (when applicable), and other regulatory agencies and guidances.	ICH GCP 4.1.3; 4.1.4; 4.10.2; 4.11 (1–3); 4.11.2; 5.17.1; 5.18.4 (o)

AEs, adverse events; GCP, good clinical practice; ICH, International Conference on Harmonization; IEC, institutional ethics committee; IRB, institutional review board; PHI, protected health information; SAEs, serious adverse events; SOPs, standard operating procedures.

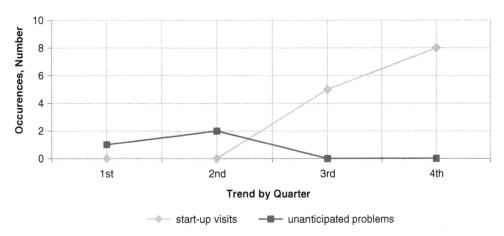

FIGURE 6.1 2013 Study start-up meetings and protocol deviations.

clinical research work is nearly identical to clinical nursing work completed as part of usual care, all nursing research staff should know the difference (subtle or major) in research requirements. Education includes specific activities that will promote adherence to data-collection rules (e.g., CRF completion) and research procedures that are consistent with the current protocol.

Research staff must have knowledge of Health Insurance Portability and Accountability Act (HIPAA) guidelines related to HSR and principles of research ethics found in the Belmont report. Organizations and institutions can subscribe to the Collaborative Institutional Training Initiative (CITI) program at the University of Miami (www.CITIprogram.org), which provides fundamental education in the form of web-based modules. Many hospital organizations and research institutions require completion of CITI courses as a prerequisite to submitting a research protocol to the IRB. The research PI is responsible for ensuring that CITI training or an alternate comprehensive human subject's research training course, per IRB criteria, is completed by all study staff before they carry out any role in the study that involves human subjects. For example, if the protocol calls for individuals in study roles to engage in research-related interactions with prospective study subjects, communication with subjects should not occur before HSR requirements are met. Knowledge gained through HSR training protects research subjects and minimizes research compliance issues related to ethics or HIPAA violations. In addition to general HSR training, the PI must carry out specific protocol training (see Table 6.3). Investigators should be able to answer "yes" to the following questions before study staff are permitted to conduct activities related to the research protocol: Is each member of the study team familiar with the purpose of the study and the protocol? Does staff have an adequate understanding of specific details of the protocol, attributes of the intervention, and use of tools or items needed to perform their assigned tasks? Are all staff competent to perform or been trained to perform tasks they are delegated? Has staff been made aware of any pertinent changes during the conduct of research

TABLE 6.3 Research Protocol Best Practices and GCP References

ISSUE PREVENTION CONSIDERATIONS	DETAILS AND RATIONALE	GCP REFERENCES
• Create a protocol number and date and list all study staff on the cover page.	• As study staff are amended, revise the cover page and create a new version number and data to keep an accurate history of protocol revisions related to personnel.	ICH GCP 8.2.2
• Maintain all versions of the protocol (signed by the PI) in the regulatory (electronic or paper) binder. If saved electronically, use a unique title so versions can be easily retrieved as needed.	• Ensures that the most recent version of the protocol is on file, and assessable to all study investigators who are actively involved in the research process.	ICH GCP 8.2.2; 8.2.7; 8.3.2
• Ensure that protocol amendments are submitted to the IRB before initiating changes in practices.	• Submit an amendment to the IRB along with the updated protocol and wait for approval *before* applying study changes. Exception: The change is to prevent an immediate hazard(s) to trial subjects.	ICH GCP 4.5.1; 4.5.2; 4.5.4
• Submit protocol amendments for studies approved as "exempt from further IRB review"	• The IRB could deem that research risks have changed and alter the status from exempt to "nonexempt." • The PI or study team cannot make a judgment about the level of risk to subjects; only the IRB can make this determination. • If the IRB electronic submittal system is closed to amendments (due to exempt status), the PI must contact the IRB to allow an amendment submission.	ICH GCP 3.3.8 (b) (c); 4.10.2

GCP, good clinical practice; ICH, International Conference on Harmonization; IRB, institutional review board; PI, principal investigator.

and received additional training as appropriate? Answers to these questions will help the PI to determine study staff training needs. Table 6.4 provides study staff training best practices and also includes general training requirements beyond the CITI human subject course. Special training requirements should be added to the research regulatory binder checklist to create consistency when educating new study team members.

The delegation of authority log is a regulatory document for drug and device studies that can be used in all research studies to show roles and responsibilities of study personnel. This best practice tracking tool includes fields for signatures and initials of all study personnel, highlights the responsibilities of each member of the study team, and lists date ranges when study team members participated. Since the delegation of authority log clarifies the roles of all team

TABLE 6.4 Study Staff Training Best Practices and GCP References

ISSUE PREVENTION CONSIDERATIONS	DETAILS AND RATIONALE	GCP REFERENCES
• Only individuals approved by the IRB can participate in the study.	• Only individuals who are trained and knowledgeable about the study should be permitted to participate as study personnel. • Keep a record of study staff training in the form of meeting minutes of in-services, e-mails, course completion printouts, and other documentation.	ICH GCP 3.3.7; 4.4.1; 5.5.1
• Only individuals approved by the IRB to participate on the study team may consent subjects, collect data, or otherwise work on the study.	• Individuals must not perform any work on the study when their approval as an investigator is pending IRB approval. Nonstudy personnel must not participate in any aspect of the study unless specified in the research protocol and IRB application, and approved by the IRB.	ICH GCP 3.3.7
• Maintain a delegation-of-responsibility log that includes each individual working on the study.	• Document roles, responsibilities, signatures of study staff, beginning and end dates of study participation, and study staff training dates.	ICH GCP 4.1.5
• Educate clinical staff who are caring for subjects involved in a research study.	• Maintain documentation of clinical research training received by clinical staff (in the regulatory files).	ICH GCP 4.2.3
• Ensure that all research staff are familiar with and adhere to pertinent research policies: IRB policies, SOPs, research compliance policies, HIPAA guidelines, data security.	• Policy awareness and adherence includes: informed consent process, investigator responsibilities, recruitment, advertising and compensation, adverse event reporting, modifications to previously approved research, reporting unanticipated problems, data handling and storage, and electronic data security.	ICH GCP 4.5.1; 4.5.2

GCP, good clinical practice; HIPAA, Health Insurance Portability and Accountability Act; ICH, International Conference on Harmonization; IRB, institutional review board; SOPs, standard operating procedures.

members, it can be referenced during quality monitoring to identify individuals who were assigned to complete specific research work, such as documenting on CRFs or applying a device on a patient to collect physiological data.

Study staff training and documentation of training has other benefits. If a study needs to be transitioned to a new nurse PI, handoff will be simpler since the new PI will have informed go-to staff resources. A seamless handoff might decrease the risk of protocol deviations during the transition period. Staff training and documentation of the functions and limits of each team member can serve to recruit team members to carry out specific research work as needed to meet timeline expectations. After IRB approval of protocol amendments, ongoing study staff training will ensure continuous compliance to new or altered requirements. Poor communication is a major cause of preventable unanticipated problems including adverse events (AEs; all risk levels), breach of confidentiality, and protocol deviations. Timely, accurate, and clear verbal and written communication reduces errors in research and improves subject safety. Study staff training enhances cohesiveness among the research team, promotes adherence to the study protocol, prevents breaches in subject confidentiality, and increases the likelihood of organized data collection procedures that might save time and improve efficiency.

CORRECTIVE AND PREVENTIVE ACTION PLANS

All PIs are responsible for handling study related issues, whether a protocol deviation, AE or serious adverse event (SAE), breach of confidentiality, or unanticipated problem involving risks. In research, the process for investigating issues, identifying root causes of issues, and preventing issues from recurring is called a corrective and preventive action plan (CAPA). Before a CAPA process is applied, the PI must establish the scope of potential harm to study subjects. If an issue appears to be an AE, major unanticipated problem or breach of confidentiality, the IRB should be notified immediately, before the development of a CAPA plan. The immediate goal of the PI should be to halt the problem. Halting new instances of the problem may involve placing the intervention or any other research procedure on hold until the present and future safety of human subjects is confirmed and potential for harm is minimized.

As the first step of the CAPA plan, a root-cause analysis will help the study team examine factors that contributed directly or indirectly to the issue. For example, while investigating an AE, the PI will need to determine if the issue only involved one or very few study subjects. Individual case studies may yield unique factors that could have contributed to the issue. The PI may find pre-existing variables in the medical record, such as previous symptoms or diagnoses (from past medical history), that occurred prior to the subject's study unit admission. Discoveries can set the precedent for amending the exclusion criteria of the protocol to prevent similar future patients from adverse harm. If the event is broader in scope, a thorough assessment may include an evaluation of subjects who experienced similar adverse reactions. It is necessary for the PI to thoroughly understand and correct the issue at its root before preventive actions can be determined.

Preventive action involves making decisions that will impact the future of the study. The goal is to prevent the previous issue from recurring. Multiple positive interventions should be considered at this step. The PI may consider the following questions:

- Do I need to amend the protocol by changing exclusion criteria so that certain types of patients are excluded from receiving the intervention?
- Do I need to change study staff responsibilities or provide re-education to study staff?
- Do I need to place the study on hold while awaiting resources that will prevent the same type of issue from recurring?

Careful and meticulous attention to choosing the right preventive action plan shows that the PI is taking ownership of issues. The goal is to protect current and future subjects from experiencing new or repeated harm.

The PI can involve study staff in the CAPA plan process by transparently sharing research issues with the team and including them in efforts to develop an overall response. It may help to interview data collectors and other study staff to receive feedback regarding observations that contributed to the issue. As a group, the study team may have an active role in providing recommendations for implementing practical, preventive solutions. Ultimately, the PI is responsible for the rollout and communication of the final CAPA plan. All staff should be trained in the new processes that encompass the new solutions. An effective CAPA plan will prevent issues from recurring in the same form or manifesting in other ways throughout the course of the study.

INFORMED-CONSENT PROCESS BEST PRACTICES

Informed-consent process best practices should reflect and supplement the regulatory policies established by the local IRB and principles found in the Belmont report and GCP. Informed consent best practices are designed to enhance subject safety, data security, and adherence to regulatory requirements (see Table 6.5). The focus of internal best practices and research quality monitoring should not duplicate the efforts of the IRB office. For example, the IRB will only approve the informed consent form (ICF) if all required elements are in place. Rather than reviewing required elements, the RQC should focus on data security measures and principles that enhance subject safety.

The PI should ensure that study personnel responsible for conducting informed-consent procedures are well trained in approaching subjects based on inclusion criteria and IRB-approved data collection methods. Also, personnel who conduct consenting procedures must have full knowledge and understanding of the protocol and be able to answer questions posed by subjects. As a best practice, the PI should document all roles related to the informed consent process in the delegation-of-authority log for the study. During an internal quality review, the RQC or research compliance reviewer will evaluate samples of completed ICFs for proper completion and check the delegation-of-authority log to ensure that study personnel responsible for informed consent match the names and signatures on consent forms. It

TABLE 6.5 Informed Consent Best Practices and GCP References

ISSUE PREVENTION CONSIDERATIONS	DETAILS AND RATIONALE	GCP REFERENCES
• Develop informed consent scripting.	• Train data collectors on the presentation of informed consent and include return demonstration as part of the process.	ICH GCP 4.2.4
• Ensure that the consent document used is the most recent IRB stamped, approved version.	• Establish a process for the removal and destruction of outdated or expired consents. *Note:* An updated, approved version of informed consent will invalidate the previous version even if the dates of use on the previous version were current.	Cleveland Clinic SOP and IRB Policy
• The person obtaining consent is assigned the role as part of the research team and approved by the IRB to participate on the study.	• At minimum, all personnel should have completed CITI course training and any other research education determined by the IRB and nursing research program. • The person handling the informed consent process should be well trained, including understanding the protocol and being able to answer subjects' questions about the study.	21 CFR 50 "The Consent Process" ICH GCP 4.1.5
• Document the informed consent process in the electronic medical record when it applies; e.g., longitudinal studies, studies with interventions (comparative designs; see topic: Data Collection Documentation, Table 6.6)	• *Note:* Minimal risk studies do *not* require documentation in the medical record. However, documentation should occur in the research file.	ICH GCP 4.8.1 AAHRPP Element III.1.F.
• The person obtaining consent must verify that the subject understands the study and voluntarily agrees to participate.	• Subjects should be given adequate time to review the informed consent and make a voluntary decision regarding participation in the study. • Exclusion criteria may include vulnerable subjects (ICH GCP 1.61).	ICH GCP 4.8.1; 4.8.3; 4.8.7
• Every research subject or LAR must sign and date his or her own consent.	• The person obtaining consent must witness the signature of the subject or LAR, then sign and date the consent in the same setting.	ICH GCP 4.8.8

(continued)

TABLE 6.5 Informed Consent Best Practices and GCP References (*continued*)

ISSUE PREVENTION CONSIDERATIONS	DETAILS AND RATIONALE	GCP REFERENCES
• Prior to study participation, the subject or subject's LAR should receive a copy of the signed and dated (by subject or LAR and consenter) written ICF and any other information provided to the subjects.	• During the trial the subject or LAR should be apprised of any updates to informed consent and receive a copy of the signed and dated consent form updates along with any changes to written information provided to subjects.	ICH GCP 4.8.11
• If a subject needs to be re-consented, the rationale must be documented in the medical record or research file.	• Reasons for re-consenting may include an amended ICF that presents new information, including new risks or new study personnel to contact for questions. • The reason for re-consent should be explained to research subjects.	ICH GCP 4.8.2; 4.8.10 (p)

CITI, Collaborative Institutional Training Initiative; GCP, good clinical practice; ICF, informed consent form; ICH, International Conference on Harmonization; IRB, institutional review board; LAR, legally authorized representative.

is expected that the IRB-approved study person who explains the research is the same individual who signed the ICF. Each IRB has its own requirements, but most ICFs have a general statement that verifies that the person obtaining consent by signature thoroughly explained the research and witnessed the subject's comprehension and willingness to participate. Adequate training of study personnel involves return demonstration of clearly and concisely explaining the research purpose, research goals, patient expectations, timeline, benefit, risks, costs, and protection of data. Provision of complete study information and confirmation of the subject's understanding prior to signing the form will minimize issues in patient adherence to interventions, data collection form completion, and follow-up participation.

During an internal quality review, the RQC or research compliance reviewer will assess the ICF to ensure it is the correct version. The IRB requires that only the current, approved ICF is used. A best practice that supports the use of the current ICF is the inclusion of a version number and/or date on the footer that corresponds with the approval usage dates. For example, if an ICF was approved by the IRB from 11/12/13 to 11/12/14, and the version number was labeled "1," the version number should be revised to "2" if the form was amended for any reason. Although it is not common to change the version number during the annual IRB study approval renewal, if changes were made to the ICF and submitted with the renewal application, the version number should be revised.

Vulnerable Subjects

PIs must ensure that vulnerable subjects have additional protections. In nursing research, it is quite common for subjects to be nurses or other health care employees of the hospital organization. Employees are considered a vulnerable population, especially when the PI is a direct or indirect supervisor or organization leader to potential or actual research subjects. Employees may fear providing data associated with a research study due to perceived repercussions associated with job hierarchy, research work expectations, communications, or feelings about the workplace, and research factors, including pressure to participate, that could be viewed as a vulnerability to undue influence or coercion. As a best practice, safeguards should be implemented to protect nurse subjects by ensuring that recruitment strategies avoid undue influence. Undue influence is minimized when research nurses who are supervisors or other leaders are excluded from face-to-face recruitment of direct reports. For example, executive nurse leaders, physicians in authority roles, nursing directors, managers, and assistant nurse managers should refrain from face-to-face recruitment of clinical nurses under their domain of influence. In addition to clinical nurses being vulnerable subjects, they may serve as patient caregivers in usual care settings to potential research subjects. They should refrain from enrolling patients in a study when they are the assigned caregivers. A research study team member should approach patients to avoid perceptions of undue influence or coercion.

Data Security

Human subjects who consent to participate in research should have assurance that optimal data security and storage practices are used. The PI must ensure that data protection is in place by locking completed ICFs and CRFs in a safe location that is inaccessible to unauthorized individuals (i.e., non-study personnel). To minimize the risk for breach of confidentiality, ICFs and CRFs should not leave the hospital organization. Exceptions are when the ICF explicitly states that a college (when a graduate student is performing research as part of course requirements) or study sponsor may have a copy. Informed consent process pitfalls that should be avoided include screening outside of (prior to or after) the study approval period, obtaining consent prior to the approved study start date, sharing incomplete information with subjects, and minimizing potential or actual risks of study participation. If a PI intends to leave the hospital organization before a research project is completed, precautions may need to be taken to ensure human subject data are not compromised. Figure 6.2 is a flowchart that provides oversight of handling of a PI request to remove data from the hospital site where research was initiated.

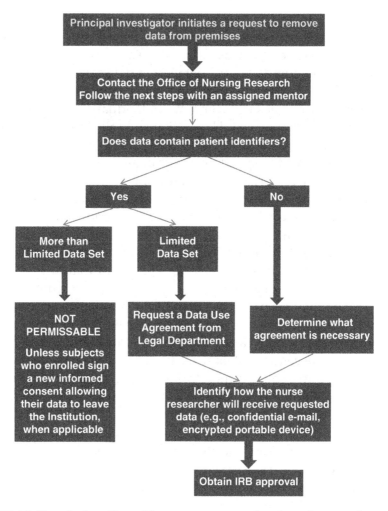

FIGURE 6.2 Steps for handling a PI request to remove data from the research premises.
IRB, institutional review board; PI, principal investigator.

Quality oversight initiatives to promote the adoption and use of best practices in the informed consent process safeguard research subjects and research teams. The PI is responsible for ensuring that systems and processes are in place before, during, and after the informed consent process is completed. Further, attention to vulnerable subjects, especially nurses and other colleagues, will create a transparent, trusting research environment that may promote future research.

DATABASE OPTIMIZATION

An adjunct of quality oversight is electronic database development and data-entry training. Nurse investigators are encouraged to set up databases for direct data entry or entry of data previously collected on paper. Database optimization training will be based on the database used. The most important factor that increases the usability of database data is that the setup must be planned based on the way data will be analyzed, not the way data appear in an electronic administrative database, a data collection form, or a valid instrument. For example, a tool may have five items that, when summed, provide information on one factor. Since the individual items are meaningless by themselves, the database would be developed to allow only the sum score (one item) to be entered. If all five items were placed in the database, the PI or a statistician would need to spend time creating a new variable that provides the sum score. If all five variables plus the sum score were developed into the database, the PI or statistician would have unnecessary data. An RQC may spend time assessing quality that is unnecessary, and statisticians may spend time creating frequencies or completing other analyses on meaningless data. Another example of optimal database setup is when you receive bloodstream infection data from your infection control department that includes the date, type of infection, source of infection, and lab draw site. For your study, all you need is "yes" or "no" regarding the presence of a bloodstream infection. After creating a database, reassess to ensure that only data that are needed for analysis are included to save time (and costs) of data entry.

A more concise database means fewer transcription errors and fewer data to assess during quality monitoring. The PI or nurse researcher mentor should always guide the RQC or other database creator in how the database should be set up to minimize time needed to prepare data for analysis. As an example, database setup for analyzing two sets of data from the same person (pre- and postdata) would use a parried t test and would look different than the setup for analyzing two sets of data from two time periods (pre- and postdata) that consist of two separate cohorts and are analyzed using an independent t test. Other important database development factors to consider are (a) how "other" responses will be handled, (b) if data on the data collection form (such as responses on a Likert-like scale) will be placed in the database as continuous data (IBM® Statistical Procedures for Social Sciences Statistics® [SPSS] uses the term "scale") or as categorical data (SPSS uses the term "ordinal"), and (c) how data with multiple response choices will be handled, since the drop-down menu in some research databases does not allow entry of all that apply and only one option can be selected. Again, not only will a statistician appreciate database development considerations, but correct inputting of variables and values of variables will save time and effort, both of which improve efficiency of resource utilization.

The RQC can assist nurses in setting up databases when the study start-up meeting is conducted, assuming the data decisions already discussed are clarified. Also, it is important for the RQC to choose the right measurement level (nominal, ordinal, interval [when applicable], or scale) based of the type of variable, as measurement level may affect the statistical tests used to analyze data. The RQC can assist a novice PI in developing a data dictionary once database development is completed. Finally, the RQC can input data with novice PIs once the first 10 cases are ready for data entry. The purpose of early data entry with support is to assess the database for functionality. Oftentimes the database must be tweaked to account for nuances in data collection. Most data nuances can be found in the first 10 cases. Once the database has been revised, the study team can work independently.

QUALITY OVERSIGHT OF DATA ENTRY

Due to human error, the data entry process presents challenges to data integrity. Even small data entry mistakes can significantly change and invalidate the statistical results of a research study (Barchard, Scott, Weintraub, & Pace, 2008). There are a variety of methods used to check and correct data after the initial data entry is complete. Of methods for checking the accuracy of data, the one-person visual check is least efficient (Barchard & Pace, 2011). To achieve a high level of quality and low error rate, PIs should select between two more efficient methods: double data entry and two-stage partner read aloud.

Double data entry is a continuous approach in which data are entered from source data (from CRFs) a second time. Double data entry is considered a state of the art approach to maintaining quality in data entry compared to other data checking methods, resulting in greater detected and corrected errors (Barchard & Pace, 2011; Barchard & Verenikina, 2013; Kawado et al., 2003). However, double entry should not be completed by the same person, as a single person may make the same error twice. In double data entry, two sets of complete data are entered before data matching is completed, and discrepancies in data are found (if errors exist) and corrected (Barchard & Verenikina, 2013). Problems may occur if the data from one entered dataset are used to match the other. Hence, the authority of correct data is the original data on the CRF or data collection instrument.

Two-stage read-aloud data cleaning is a post-quality check in which one person reads source data from CRFs out loud while a second person checks the completed database for correctness of entry. Any data discrepancy will lead to a correction in the database. Prior to initiating the read-aloud method, frequencies of all data should be obtained and obvious missing data and data errors should be corrected; for example, inaccurate subject ages, dates, and value entries that were not established as accurate values in the data dictionary. Since read-aloud data cleaning should only be considered following the implementation of quality controls that reduce mistakes of single (original) data entry, there may be a low acceptable error rate when using the two-stage read-aloud data cleaning method (Buchele, Och, Bolte, & Weiland, 2005), unless error rates are counted after the first step is completed. PIs may prefer the two-stage read-aloud method because it is less time consuming and uses fewer resources compared to the double data entry process (Buchele et al., 2005). Optimal quality and accuracy of outcomes are the main focus behind data check decisions. At the Cleveland Clinic, we use the two-stage read-aloud data cleaning method most often and have very high standards for quality. The process involves assessing 20% of all cases, no matter how large the data set is. If data cleaning accuracy (where each mistake is counted as one error) is less than 98%, 50% of all cases are reviewed. If data cleaning accuracy in 50% of cases is below 98%, then 100% of data is assessed for quality before data are ready for statistical analysis.

If systematic errors are discovered during data checks, the PI should be consulted. The PI may ask questions to identify the root cause of the errors: Was there a particular data entry person who consistently inserted the wrong variable response or misinterpreted information on CRFs? Did all data collectors misinterpret a data point on the CRF? Did a data entry person miss a data entry point and the remainder of data entry for the case was inaccurate? Answers to questions will determine an action plan. For data verification purposes, in the Cleveland Clinic nursing research program, a data point is created in the database for the data entry person's initials for each CRF. If one person persistently entered incorrect responses to one or more data points, all data for that data point entered by that person will need to be checked. When values are misinterpreted or fall outside of the range of acceptable values, information can be checked against the CRF or other secondary source data. If values are incorrect on various forms of source data, validity of the data must be challenged (Day, Fayers, & Harvey, 1998). If primary source data are available (medical record or laboratory data), CRF corrections should be made before corrections are applied in the database. The PI must use discretion regarding how to handle systematic data issues and consider the effect of quality measures on data analysis and research findings.

There are multiple methods for enhancing the quality of original (single) data entry. Methods include restricting cell content to prevent spelling errors, setting value limits, comparing adjacent entries to detect major discrepancies, comparing the sample size with the number of units in the database, and performing logical checks to detect when values are mistakenly copied into other cells (Buchele et al., 2005).The PI should ensure that training of data collectors and data entry staff includes standard expectations of CRF completion. Data collectors need to develop a system for monitoring completed CRFs; especially early after data collection begins and whenever new study team members are added. Education that prevents interpretation problems promotes a high degree of data quality and integrity.

Data quality in the data collection and entry processes means that data should be accurate, legible, complete, and contemporaneous (recorded at the time the activity occurs), original, and attributed to the person who generated the data (*Handbook for Good Clinical Research Practice, Guidance for Implementation*, World Health Organization, 2005). Data integrity refers to the soundness of the entire body of data so that data are credible, internally consistent, and verifiable. Data quality and integrity are achieved when each piece of data is carefully collected in harmony with the study protocol and procedures, and subsequently handled so that the characteristics of the original data are preserved in transcription and interpretation. When efforts are directed to optimization of data collection and single data entry, selection of the type of data check will have less of an impact on the overall soundness and quality of the data set.

QUALITY EFFORTS TO MINIMIZE MISSING AND INACCURATE DATA

Missing data on subject-administered tools/instruments or inaccurately completed CRFs can hamper the accuracy of analysis. To decrease the incidence of missing and inaccurate data, PIs should train the study team in data collection. If several study staff are data collectors, there is an added burden of reliability of data collected among the study staff. The PI is responsible for monitoring the quality of data collected.

Some tips are available to increase accuracy and completeness of data collected. Meet regularly with the study team, preferably together, and discuss issues and solutions (see Table 6.6). When data points are missing or inaccurate, the following questions should lead to group discussion: Why was the data point missed or inaccurate? Was the omission or inaccuracy an oversight (random error)? Was the omission or inaccuracy observed repeatedly (systematic error)? If random error is discovered, one action is to review CRFs for completion at the time of data collection, whenever possible. Use a spiral notebook or electronic site to record random errors and decisions made about how to handle them, so that other random errors can be adjudicated using the same solutions. If the errors found are systematic, the PI should retrain the study team and possibly limit the number of data collectors. Quality monitoring of data collected should occur regularly until the PI is assured of high-quality data collection. At the Cleveland Clinic, we ask nurses collecting data to place their initials on the form so we can quickly identify those who are very accurate and those who might need retraining or re-assignment. Finally, for each variable, all possible response options must be exhausted, so that subjects are not confronted with having to select between options that are not good answers, and ultimately choose to leave the item blank. If the possible response options are a long list, "other" can be used, but "not applicable" may also be the best response. Completeness of response options will not be an issue when valid, reliable instruments are used. Novice PIs should discuss data collection forms with a nurse researcher mentor to ensure investigator-developed forms are complete and less likely to lead to omission and inaccurate data entries/responses. Table 6.6 presents data collection documentation best practices and examples of systematic adjudication of common missing data or inaccurate variable values. Table 6.7 provides best practices related to preparing data for data analysis.

TABLE 6.6 Data Collection Documentation Best Practices and GCP References

ISSUE PREVENTION CONSIDERATIONS	DETAILS AND RATIONALE	GCP REFERENCES
• Informed consent process: In the medical record, investigator will document that voluntariness was explained along with inclusion and exclusion criteria, intervention delivery, and potential risks, and that subject agreement was confirmed.	• Researchers should apply the general rule: "If it was not documented, it was not done."	ICH GCP 1.28; 4.8.1 AAHRPP Element III.1.F.
• CRFs should match the protocol exactly. Instruments should be valid and reliable before being used in a research study.	• Investigator-developed instruments must be examined for face and content validity, at minimum, before use in a research study.	ICH GCP 4.9.4
• Data correction education should be provided to all study staff for both electronic and paper corrections. • PIs and sponsors (if applicable) should provide written procedures to ensure that changes or corrections in CRFs by designated study staff are documented, necessary, and endorsed by the investigator.	• Any paper-based CRF data corrections are made using a single strike through the original entry, not obscuring the original entry. Corrections should be made with blue or black ink, and the person making the corrections should place the date and his or her initials next to the corrected entry.	ICH GCP 4.9.1; 4.9.3
• Corrections made to a CRF should be explained (if necessary) and should not obscure the original entry. This applies to written and electronic corrections.	• For an accurate reference of the data collector who made corrections, initials of all data collectors should be signed on the delegation of authority log.	ICH GCP 4.9.3; 5.18.4 (n)

• Adjudication of data should be systematic whenever possible.	• Examples of data adjudication:
	  ▪ Missing the event year: Select the most plausible year based on known facts surrounding the event. If there is a range of possible years, select the median value
	  ▪ Missing month: select July
	  ▪ Missing day-of-month: select 15th of month
	  ▪ In multiple choice item, if multiple responses were selected when only one response was required, select the first option selected
	  ▪ If multiple choice item is a knowledge survey, and more than one response was selected, if the "right answer" was selected, accept that response, even if wrong answers were also selected
		Not applicable

CRF, case report form; GCP, good clinical practice; ICH, International Conference on Harmonization; PI, principal investigator.

TABLE 6.7 Best Practices that Enhance Data Analysis Capabilities

BEST PRACTICE	RATIONALE	REMEDY	EXAMPLES
When possible, numerically code responses (create values for variables) to provide consistent data entry.	Since capitalization and spelling differences are read as distinct responses, numbers are easier to make uniform.	Provide numerically coded responses, with a key to translate the numbers to meaningful responses.	It is a convention to treat 0 = No and 1 = Yes. Rather than entering complications text, "no" complications may be coded as 0 and "yes," complications may be coded as 1.
Do not include comments as fields to be analyzed.	Searching text can be slow and difficult.	If there is important information to be used in a comment, then create a separate column for that measure.	If interested in whether encounter notes recommended a diet change, create a separate field for "diet change" with Yes/No response options.
For numeric measures, collect the actual measure and categorize later, if necessary.	It is easier to collapse levels into bigger categories, but not possible to split into smaller levels.	Avoid capturing numeric measures in category groups unless it is certain that the grouping is final.	If age groups will be analyzed as pediatric vs. adult, collect the actual age, then create cut points for splitting patients on age (e.g., <18 and 18 or older).
Include one piece of information in each data field.	Most analyses will require separation, and inclusion of special characters can cause problems.	Separate related fields into multiple columns.	Instead of capturing blood pressure as 120/80 in a single field, capture systolic and diastolic measures as separate columns.
Collect *dates* in a consistent format.	Dates (especially two-digit years) can be read differently depending on the program.	Make sure that dates are entered in a consistent format, and include four-digit years to avoid problems on import.	Dates such as 3/12/19 can represent multiple possible dates. Use four-digit years and make sure months and days are consistent.

VOICE OF A BIOSTATISTICIAN: PREPARING DATA FOR ANALYSIS

James F. Bena, MS
Lead Biostatistician, Quantitative Health Sciences, Cleveland Clinic Health System, Cleveland, Ohio

Preparing data for analysis is often one of the most underappreciated aspects of statistical analysis. It is common for data collected during a study not to match the format needed for analysis. In most

(continued)

VOICE OF A BIOSTATISTICIAN (*continued*)

cases, changes required can be made by the person performing the analysis after data are imported into a statistical program for analysis. However, researchers should not rely on being able to make changes after data collection is complete. Ideally, common issues should be considered up front and handled early in the data collection phase. The following provides some suggestions to help make the transition from data collection to analysis as smooth as possible.

Electronic database programs can help format data in a way best suited for analysis. Develop the database as the study begins, and check to be sure that "limits" are set to ensure that data entries are consistent and accurate (e.g., a value has a specific cut-off limit or range to be considered accurate). Spreadsheet software not developed for research data collection purposes may allow data deletion, data changes, and data sorting in ways that make it very difficult to recover the original data.

Even when using a research database program, care must be taken to make sure data are captured in a way that best allows for analysis. Since statistical software is often quite limited in how data are viewed, planning for data collection can provide the best results. In particular, text responses can be difficult to handle since most statistical programs treat variations in spelling and capitalization of text as different responses. For example, if gender responses included "m," "M," "Male," "male," and "MALE," each would be treated as different responses, rather than collectively being treated as males. Finding gender entry errors may be easily done, but for other measures, such as diagnoses and medications, it can be quite challenging to properly find all possible options for data entry and classify them correctly.

Similarly, extracting text can be a challenge using statistical software, even though most programs have searching capabilities. If text from operative notes were included as a field in the database, and researchers wanted to know if complications were listed in the notes, it would be possible to search the operative note field, and treat any match of the word "complication" as a "yes" response. However, data entry personnel would need to know, up front, to use the term "complication" consistently and not use other terms with the same meaning. If a note contained the phrase "no complications observed," the software would find a match for the word of interest and would incorrectly say "yes" to complication. For that reason, it is best to capture key measures as separate fields rather

(*continued*)

> ### VOICE OF A BIOSTATISTICIAN (*continued*)
>
> than relying on the computer to identify them correctly from text fields. Best practices and tips for data collection in preparation for data analysis are captured in Table 6.7.
>
> In summary, setting up a research database (using the right programs) at the beginning of your study, being consistent in data collection, and working with a statistician and nursing research mentor to make sure that data collection methods are ideal will lead to the most timely and best results for performing the analysis when the study is completed.

QUALITY EXPECTATIONS FOR EDUCATION OF NURSE INVESTIGATORS AND VISITING RESEARCHERS

Since clinical hospital-based nurse investigators are often novices in research processes, they may not have ever been educated in research ethics, human subjects protection, patient safety from fraud or misconduct, and other elements of GCP (Gupta, 2013). Additionally, visiting researchers are required to meet the same research education requirements as hospital-based nurse investigators. Visiting researchers are generally nurses who (a) work for the hospital organization and are completing research as part of a college commitment—thus, research is not work related (even if research findings would benefit nursing departments, nursing units where the visiting researcher is employed, or the hospital organization); or (b) do not work for the hospital organization, but desire to *assist hospital organization nurses* in an already IRB-approved research study to gain practical experience as a part of a graduate program research assignment or hospital exchange program, or *initiate and implement a research study* within the organization, using subjects available within the hospital organization. Visiting researchers who are expert nurse researchers from local academic settings may understand research ethics, human subjects protection, patient safety from fraud or misconduct, and other elements of GCP. Further, they have experience writing scientifically sound research protocols that include optimal protection of human subjects and may have previously received grant funding; however, they may experience increased research quality monitoring due to lack of familiarity with hospital organization SOPs and nonemployee status.

When novice or experienced nurse investigators or visiting researchers are involved in nursing research but are unfamiliar with hospital organization research policies, quality monitoring is required and may need to be routinely applied to minimize and manage potential compliance risks to procedural standards. Development and enforcement of visiting researcher policies,

SOPs, and contracts (e.g., a data use agreement) ensures that protections are in place for research subjects (patients and hospital staff), and for subjects' privileged data.

The nursing research program leader must develop an action plan that includes pre-research start-up, research conduct, and data management and storage components. During the pre-research start-up phase, hospital organization nurse investigators and visiting researchers must fulfill requirements that ensure they understand guidelines related to GCP and protection of human subjects prior to submission to the IRB. Training includes hospital organization education courses and modules for Human Subjects Research (HSR) that promotes research quality and public trust. The CITI HSR program commonly used by hospitals has a biomedical focus. There is also a course that involves social, behavioral, and educational disciplines, all three of which are common themes of nursing research (National Research Council, 2011). The CITI HSR program courses include content on the historical development of human subjects protections, and regulatory and ethical issues. In addition to HSR, nurses need to understand research GCP content themes, such as understanding and obtaining informed consent, developing and maintaining a regulatory binder, and reporting unanticipated problems, adverse effects, and serious adverse effects (see Table 6.8). A checklist or website can be used to track completion of education elements, training, and paperwork. Further, for

TABLE 6.8 Research Education to Promote GCP

OPTION A—LIVE COURSE: 4.5 HOUR INVESTIGATOR EDUCATION	OPTION B—SELF-STUDY: THREE EDUCATION MODULES WITH A COMBINED 30-ITEM QUIZ; REVIEWED BY A NURSE RESEARCHER*
• Humans subjects research process • Conflict of interest • Database and clinical data management • Legal agreements • Trial budgeting and billing compliance • Advanced trial design and protocol writing • IRB submission • Application and review criteria • Informed consent document • Informed consent process • Unanticipated problems–deviations • AEs/SAEs	**Module 1: The Informed Consent Process** • Documentation requirements • Elements of informed consent and examples • Assessing subject comprehension **Module 2: Regulatory Binder Essentials** • Identification of necessary regulatory documents • Binder organization and standardization • Tools and templates to complete essential regulatory files • Ongoing maintenance of regulatory records **Module 3: Understanding Unanticipated Problems and AEs/SAEs** • Correctly identifying events that require reporting • Preventing the occurrence of unanticipated problems • Review of the IRB reporting form • Case studies; best practices

*The 30-item quiz in Option B is reviewed by a doctorate-prepared nurse researcher, and responses are discussed directly with the nurse investigator or visiting researcher.

AEs, adverse events; IRB, institutional review board; SAEs, serious adverse events.

visiting researchers, quality of research conduct, data management, and storage components should match expectations of all hospital organization nurse research investigators.

From an ethics standpoint and based on state work rules, visiting researchers who are also hospital organization nurse employees (working on a college degree) must be identified as visiting researchers when completing research work to meet college requirements (college education and paid work must remain separate). Temporary (volunteer) badges usually have a different appearance. A temporary badge visibly increases the awareness of nurse colleagues and leaders to employed nurses' participation in research work as a visiting researcher. Clear identification of a visiting researcher may minimize potential conflicts related to time spent completing research as opposed to work duties that are part of paid employment.

TABLE 6.9 HIPAA Privacy Rule, Two Methods

REQUIREMENTS FOR DE-IDENTIFICATION OF PHI	
"EXPERT DETERMINATION" METHOD	"SAFE HARBOR" METHOD

Health information is not individually identifiable health information only if:
• A person with appropriate knowledge of and experience with generally accepted statistical and scientific principles and methods for rendering information not individually identifiable who is applying such principles and methods:
   ■ Determines that the risk is very small that information could be used alone or in combination with other reasonably available information by an anticipated recipient to identify an individual who is a subject of the information; and
   ■ Documents the methods and results of the analysis that justify such determination.
	Completely Removed Identifiers:
	• Names
	• Geographical subdivisions smaller than a state: street address, city, county, precinct, zip code
	• Elements of dates (except year) for dates directly related to a person, including birth, admission or discharge dates; date of death; and all ages over 89 years and all elements of dates that indicate age of 90 years and older, unless a single category of age, 90 years or older is used
	• Phone and fax numbers
	• Electronic mail addresses
	• Social Security numbers
	• Medical record numbers
	• Health plan beneficiary numbers
	• Account numbers
	• Certificate/license numbers
	• Vehicle identifiers and serial numbers, including license plate numbers
	• Device identifiers and serial numbers
	• Web universal resource locators (URLs)
	• Internet protocol (IP) address numbers
	• Biometric identifiers, including finger and voice prints
	• Full-face photographic images and any comparable images
	• Any unique identifying number, characteristic, or code (specific to the person; e.g., tattoos)

HIPAA, Health Insurance Portability and Accountability Act; IP, Internet protocol; PHI, protected health information; URL, universal resource locator.

Adapted from U.S. Department of Health and Human Services (2012).

When visiting researchers are PIs, the type of data collected will dictate the level of quality monitoring required during data collection and management. For PHI with identifiers (PHI; see Table 6.9), the hospital organization nurse investigator and nurse researcher coach or mentor must ask the following questions: How will the data with PHI be used? Will PHI data remain on site or will it be shared externally? Will data be shared as de-identified data (PHI factors removed)? A data-use agreement sets restrictions on the type of data that can be shared and how data will be used by external parties. All nurse investigators should safeguard traveling with PHI data by protecting subject files. An encrypted electronic storage device should be used to store and travel with electronic data. Moreover, data should be locked in a file cabinet or electronic database when not in use.

SUMMARY

Communication of quality objectives and implementation of best practices will enhance nursing research processes. Quality issues are expected whenever there is human involvement in research practices. However, repetitive education and the customization of elements of quality oversight will enhance data integrity and promote a nursing research program culture of excellence. Education in comprehensive quality management empowers nurses conducting research to successfully maintain quality on every level of the research process. Study start-up meetings, research compliance awareness, study staff training, and data optimization all contribute to a high-quality nursing research program. When reliable quality efforts are employed to prevent and minimize occurrence of issues, the nursing research program benefits from optimal use of time and personnel.

REFERENCES

Barchard, K., Scott, J., Weintraub, D., & Pace, L. (2008, August). *Better data entry: Double entry is superior to visual checking*. Paper presented at the American Psychological Association Annual Convention, Boston, MA.

Barchard, K., & Pace, L. (2011). Preventing human error: The impact of data entry methods on data accuracy and statistical results. *Computers in Human Behavior, 27,* 1834–1839. doi: 10.1016/j.chb.2011.04.004

Barchard, K., & Verenikina, Y. (2013). Improving data accuracy: Selecting the best data technique. *Computers in Human Behavior, 29*(5), 1917–1922. doi: 10.1016/j.chb.2013 .02.021

Buchele, G., Och, B., Bolte, G., & Weiland, S. K. (2005). Single vs. double data entry. *Epidemiology 16*(1), 130–131. doi: 10.1097/01.ede.0000147166.24478.f4

Day, S., Fayers, P., & Harvey, D. (1998). Double data entry: What value, what price? *Controlled Clinical Trials, 19* (1), 15–24. doi: 10.1016/S0197-2456(97)00096-2

Gupta, A. (2013). Fraud and misconduct in clinical research: A concern. *Perspectives in Clinical Research, 4*(2), 144–147. doi: 10.4103/2229-3485.111800

Kawado, M., Hinotsu, S., Matsuyama, Y., Yamaguchi, T., Hashimoto, S., & Ohashi, Y. (2003). A comparison of error detection rates between the reading aloud method and double data entry method. *Controlled Clinical Trials, 24* (5): 560–569.

National Research Council. (2011). *Research Training in the Biomedical, Behavioral, and Clinical Research Sciences.* Washington, DC: The National Academies Press. https://grants.nih.gov/training/Research_Training_Biomedical.pdf

The Office of Inspector General of the U.S. Department of Health and Human Services and The American Health Lawyers Association. (2007). *Corporate Responsibility and Health Care Quality: A Resource for Health Care Boards of Directors.* Retrieved from https://oig.hhs.gov/fraud/docs/complianceguidance/CorporateResponsibilityFinal%209-4-07.pdf

U.S. Department of Health and Human Services. (2012). *Guidance regarding methods for de-identification of protected health information in accordance with the Health Insurance Portability and Accountability Act (HIPAA) privacy rule.* Retrieved from http://www.hhs.gov/ocr/privacy/hipaa/understanding/coveredentities/De-identification/guidance.html

U.S. Department of Health and Human Services Food and Drug Administration. (Procedural, 2009). *Guidance for Industry: Investigator Responsibilities—Protecting the Rights, Safety, and Welfare of Study Subjects.* Retrieved from http://www.fda.gov/downloads/Drugs/.../Guidances/UCM187772.pdf

World Health Organization. (2002). *Handbook for Good Clinical Research Practice (GCP): Guidance for Implementation.* Geneva, Switzerland: World Health Organization. Retrieved from http://apps.who.int/prequal/info_general/documents/GCP/gcp1.pdf

Esther I. Bernhofer

7

MOVING PAST TRADITIONAL NURSING RESEARCH PROGRAM BARRIERS TOWARD SUCCESS

Despite the growing recognition of the importance of clinical nurses conducting research in hospitals, barriers to actively initiating, completing, and publishing original clinical nurse-led research remains (Tanner & Hale, 2002); Table 1.1 in Chapter 1 lists many barriers cited in the literature. Traditional barriers can be categorized into three clusters: (a) problems with nursing research visibility/priority, (b) finding nursing time and money for research, and (c) education regarding conducting, disseminating, and translating research. Beyond having nurse researcher support, movement toward a vibrant, successful program—as evidenced by improved patient satisfaction, quality of care, safety, clinical outcomes, nurse efficiencies, and cost savings—involves dealing with potential and actual barriers, even if they initially appear insurmountable. Fortunately, there are effective strategies that can be implemented by a motivated nursing research team.

The purpose of this chapter is to provide examples of programs and services beyond the foundational elements discussed in Chapter 2 and global resources discussed in Chapter 3 that can be used to overcome traditional nursing research barriers. In this chapter, it is assumed that at least one doctorate-prepared nurse researcher is available to facilitate research opportunities and educate nurses about research and evidence-based practice.

INCREASING NURSING RESEARCH PROGRAM VISIBILITY

The visibility of a nursing research program is essential to its establishment and growth. To be valued, nursing research must be visible at all levels—by novice and experienced nurses, by nurse managers and leaders, and by the interprofessional teams with which nursing collaborates. Current programs may already exist in an institution and can be used to promote nursing research, increasing its visibility throughout the hospital organization system. Spending time in activities that make research visible will result in a positive cycle of nursing leadership's appreciation of the value of research and of making time and education available for research.

VOICE OF A NURSE RESEARCHER

Cynthia Bautista, PhD, RN, CNRN, SCRN, CCNS, ACNS-BC, FNCS
Neuroscience Clinical Nurse Specialist, Yale–New Haven Hospital,
New Haven, Connecticut

As a doctorate-prepared (PhD) clinical nurse specialist who facilitates evidence-based practice at my institution, I have many opportunities to coach/assist staff nurses to begin their first research study. There are a variety of reasons that nurses seek to conduct research. Most of the time it is for school, as nurses work on advanced degrees. Another reason is appreciation for Magnet® designation, and a need to facilitate engagement in nursing research by staff nurses at the bedside. I was asked to facilitate staff nurses in research. We use the *Focus Group Method* by Marianne Chulay to identify a practical research question that can then be studied (Chulay, 2006). Using the Chulay method allows staff nurses to create a study that focuses on their daily work.

Nursing leadership allows staff nurses to create protocols, collect and analyze data, and present study results during regular shift time. Staff nurses can come to work 1 hour before their shift or stay 1 hour after their shift to complete research work.

Nursing Research Can Be Fun and Doable

Increasing the priority status and visibility of nursing research throughout the institution may be a critical step in increasing the number and quality of nursing research projects, but unless the clinical nurse perceives that conducting research can be a great experience, even *fun*, it may be difficult to convince busy clinicians to take time and extra effort to start a research study. Furthermore, many nurses, at all levels, may consider clinical research a non-doable venture, since it requires knowledge and resources beyond their expertise. Therefore, when completing visibility efforts in the hospital organization, the enjoyment of investigation, the thrill of discovery, and the understanding that research *can be completed* by clinical nurses (with mentorship and resources) must be emphasized. Nurses must be encouraged to pursue their research questions in areas of interest and expertise, and in populations of available subjects. Frustration will decrease and excitement will increase when projects are designed to be relatively simple (at least for first-time projects), reasonable in scale, planned so that data collection fits with practice routines, and free of political landmines. When nursing research comes to life with nurses who are converted believers that research is fun and fulfilling, word will spread to their colleagues and the visibility and priority of nursing research will blossom.

Nursing Research Brochure

No matter how small or large the hospital organization, most are complex. Many clinical nurses fully understand their clinical roles but are completely unaware of opportunities and resources in nursing research within their hospital. A nursing research brochure can create new awareness of existing nursing research structures, systems, and processes. It can be mailed to individual nurses' homes, placed on large bulletin boards, and distributed at educational sessions and hospital-based clinical conferences. The brochure can become an ongoing reminder to nurse managers and leaders about services and can be delivered to individual nurses during an annual performance review, nurse residency graduation, and other events in which professional development and nurse leadership themes are fostered.

Nursing Research Newsletter

A regularly published nursing research newsletter reminds clinicians and those in nursing leadership of ongoing nursing research and its importance, thus keeping nursing research visible as a priority of the institution. Regular columns and features of the newsletter could include showcasing new research projects in process that have recently received institutional review board (IRB) approval; completed research projects; local, regional, and national presentations of nursing research completed by hospital nurses; and recent publication references. Segments or regular columns could include interviews with principal investigators, statisticians, and other research team members. Other ideas for interesting columns include statistics, proposal writing tips, available/ new resources, or "ask the researcher." The newsletter could also be an avenue for promoting less-known resources, research education events, conferences, internal and external research funding awards, and deadlines. Providing paper copies of the newsletter to all nurses is a traditional format for distribution. Making it available electronically creates far greater reach to more nurses and administrators in a timely and cost-effective manner.

Columns That Share Research Activities
By sharing nurses' achievements in research—such as newly approved proposal applications (title, research nurses involved, units involved, and a short description) or completed and published research projects—other clinical nurses will be more aware of ongoing research and may wish to get involved in a current project or develop their own.

Columns That Share Local, Regional, and National Presentations
of Nursing Research
Nurses who complete a research project are obligated to disseminate their findings and often do so by presenting a poster or paper (oral presentation) at local, regional, or national conferences. Photographs and short descriptions of research that was presented, including information on the nurse principal investigator, can be encouraging to nurse clinicians who are considering pursuing research.

Columns That List Recent Peer-Reviewed Publications and Media Attention
Publication of original research in a peer-reviewed scientific journal is an essential part of any investigative project. Once published, media groups (hospital-based, local community, regional, or national) may pick up a story about research findings and help spread the findings more globally. It is very exciting for clinical nurses to see their names as authors in highly esteemed journals. Keeping track of publications and media attention in a newsletter becomes a source of well-earned pride for the nursing research team and a goal for other clinical nurses interested in research.

Columns Featuring Research Resources
Support in research is important. Newsletter communication of access to statisticians, librarians, funding opportunities, interdisciplinary research experts, and other currently available resources can incentivize nurses to initiate a research project. Communication of resources provides an easy-to-find source of support opportunities for new research nurses and may be a sought-after, go-to newsletter feature.

Unit Based Journal Clubs

Often, a journal club is created for clinical nurses, as part of the commitment of the leadership of a nursing unit to provide ongoing professional education and discussion of relevant nursing practices. Journal clubs can be structured in various ways to accommodate busy nurses' schedules (Aiello-Laws, Clark, Steele-Moses, Jardine, & McGee, 2010; Westlake et al., 2014). Clubs should include a designated leader and an agenda that includes scientific literature on topics of interest to nurses. Members of the journal club can decide on whether they should meet for discussions on a monthly, quarterly, or other convenient basis. Articles for discussion can be provided to members in electronic or print formats. Further incentive for journal club participation may include obtaining nursing continuing education hours for time spent reading and discussing the literature. If the leader is not well-versed in reviewing and critiquing scientific literature, a nurse researcher can provide valuable guidance. A review of published research may stimulate interest in initiating research, especially if there were unanswered clinical questions raised during discussions.

Official and Informal Presentations of Completed Research

An effective motivator for embarking on and/or completing any research project is to see how others completed project work. Embarking on and completing a full research study is often a daunting and rigorous task and should be celebrated. Nurses who complete research should be encouraged to present their findings at the unit level and at department and leadership meetings. Formal and informal presentations celebrate research teams' accomplishments, disseminate findings, and increase nursing research visibility among clinical nurses and nursing leadership, further establishing the importance and doability of conducting nursing research. Presentation methods include poster discussions, short talks on the nursing unit during a huddle or staff/council meeting, and lunchtime discussions. A slide presentation can be prepared for leadership and will introduce nurses to the art of delivering professional presentations.

Clinical/Career/Professional Ladder Program Progression

Whether called a clinical ladder, career ladder, professional ladder, or other name (herein referred to as the *clinical ladder*), many hospitals reward clinical nurses for professional and educational advancement and demonstrated clinical excellence in nursing by movement up a status ladder (Donley & Flaherty, 2008). Nursing status designations are generally conveyed in titling, with higher numbers associated with higher professional level achieved (Cleveland Clinic, 2014; Duke Nursing, 2014; Penn State Hershey, 2014). Higher status may be associated with a monetary reward, special recognition, or both. Hospital requirements for advancing in the clinical ladder vary by hospital organization, and should include an advancing track for nursing research. Since nursing research work generally requires research and human subject protection education, and may take multiple years to complete, clinical ladder points should reflect the multiple stages of the research process (proposal development, IRB approval, data collection, analysis, dissemination, and translation) and the complexity of the work. In that way, nurses are appropriately rewarded when they complete milestones and may be more excited to take on a research project as part of clinical ladder progression. A research track can be included in all levels of the clinical ladder beyond the novice level. Including research at low levels of the track helps establish research as an important nursing structure and creates enthusiasm for advancing nursing science among early career nurses. Ultimately, visibility of nursing research at lower levels of the clinical ladder sends a message that research is valued by nursing, and that expert nurse status is not needed to initiate a research study.

Professional Development Programs

Many nursing departments within hospitals have well-designed professional development programs in place that provide clinical nurses with opportunities to expand knowledge and improve clinical skills (LoBiondo-Wood & Haber, 2013). In addition, professional development includes understanding the state of the science in nursing by acquiring and translating new knowledge, contributing to nursing science through research, and implementing evidence-based practice (American Nurses Association, 2010). Nursing research, therefore, should be incorporated into existing nursing professional development programs. This can be done in ways that add very little cost and have the potential to engage nurses in understanding the importance of research possibilities and the resources that are available. Nursing research councils often promote professional development of nurses and are discussed in Chapter 4. Development and promotion of research education opportunities increase the overall visibility of nursing research and may spur excitement for and growth in nurses' value of research.

Nurse Residency Program Graduation Celebrations

Many new nurse residency programs are 1 year in length and include a graduation session/celebration. During the residency program, new nurses are focused on tasks, critical thinking, and applying nursing practices (patient care planning, patient education, care coordination, and discharge and transition care services) and generally do not consider professional growth beyond integration on the nursing unit and within the hospital organization. At graduation, however, nurses should be ready to be introduced to nursing research resources within the hospital. Readiness to seek new knowledge through research should not be underestimated among nurses who have spent time in a nurse residency program. A 15-minute presentation that focuses on why nursing research implementation is important to the profession, to clients served, to the nursing department and hospital, and also to personal professional growth, may spark interest and excitement. During the short presentation, nurses may be inspired by the passion exhibited by the nurse researcher presenter, especially if the presentation includes an acknowledgment that most nurses who began the research journey were true novices, and that resources and support are available during every step of the process.

Nursing Leadership Annual Performance Review

Clinical nurses and nursing leaders are subject to annual (or even semi-annual) performance reviews that may include an evaluation on how specific organizational and nursing department goals were met. When organization or department goals include a report of completion and dissemination of nurse-led research, nursing research becomes increasingly important to nurse leaders and their direct reports, such as clinical nurse specialists (CNSs), nurse practitioners, nurse managers, or clinical directors. Including a specific job expectation—for example, evidence of at least one research project in progress or completed per year, per nursing leader on behalf of their team—creates an expectation that nursing team members should actively engage in nursing research. Nursing research will then be discussed among nurse leaders and their direct reports. Clinical nurses will be encouraged to pursue research and will be provided with time and resources.

ALLOCATING TIME AND MONEY FOR NURSING RESEARCH

The ubiquitous staffing and budgetary constraints of clinical nurses creates challenges to conducting clinical nursing research, especially when time must be taken away from direct patient care to plan and carry out research work (Saladino & Gosselin, 2014). There are no easy ways to make time and money appear for research projects led by clinical nurses, but creative use of structures that are already in place in the hospital organization may enable research work to become a natural part of a nursing department's scheduling and budget considerations.

VOICES OF NURSE RESEARCHERS

Karen Johnson, PhD, RN
Director, Nursing Research, Banner Health, Phoenix, Arizona

Without a doubt, getting clinical nurses the time to complete a research study is the biggest barrier. For the most part, it seems it is manager driven. That is why getting manager/leadership support of projects before they even begin is key. Most managers do support giving staff 4 hours per week (so they don't go into overtime). If at all possible, based on study design, it is always best to have studies and data collection that are part of routine clinical practice. We have staff on "light duty" help with data collection. We've even used our hospital volunteers to help with studies when we ask patients to complete surveys. Due to time constraints, we require our principal investigators (PIs) to be master's-prepared as many of them are in exempt positions.

David Pickham, PhD, RN
Director of Research, Patient Care Services, Stanford Health Care, Stanford, California

Time is by far the biggest challenge for clinical nurses developing research. The answer to this is very difficult. We could look to other professions for a model of time management, but other professions do not have the same working environment as nurses. Physicians negotiate research time into their positions with expectations of productivity and tenure. Research is valuable for physicians and they dedicate time on and off work to pursue it. I believe we need to position nursing research in the same way. We need to make it a key component of a nurse's role, combine it within evaluations, and link it to career ladders. That way research will no longer be a sideshow, but an integral component that nurses need to perform to advance their professional role. Until this time, however, release time continues to have to be negotiated on a case-by-case basis.

Nursing Research Internship

Nursing research internships are defined here as internally funded research programs that are awarded to clinical nurses for a specific period of time. The program has a defined timeline in terms of milestones completed and outcome expectations, minimal requirements for application, and clear expectations about resources used to support completion of the internship; for example, the number of hours per pay period or month that are devoted to research. In some programs, nurses cannot apply individually; they must be part of a team that will work on a project together. The advantage of a team approach is that if one person leaves the team, the research will continue to completion. A disadvantage of a team approach is that an individual nurse with a great research question may not be able to find other clinical nurses who support the research. Hospital organizations need to determine the number of internships they can support each year. To be cost-efficient, the number of internships should be based on availability of doctorate-prepared nurse researchers to coach nurses through the research process and the amount of funding available to support time away from clinical care. Clinical nurses would be discouraged if research time was constantly removed due to staffing issues; thus, an internship program works best when the hospital organization and nursing leadership make a commitment to the program and maintain the prespecified timeline and outcome expectations.

Grant and Funding Acquisition

Nursing research work is costly, primarily for time away from clinical nursing work to develop and implement research, interpret findings, and translate and disseminate results. In addition, there are costs for biostatistician time and time away from the hospital to present research externally. Nurse investigators may be confronted with how to pay for their time spent in research work and also for supplies, equipment, and consultation fees.

Many research grants are available to nurses. Obtaining grant funding is often the best, and may be the only way that research can be completed, even if the nursing department has dedicated operating funds available for research processes and a dedicated nursing research program. There is a saying regarding state lotteries: *You can't win if you don't play*. In research, the same philosophy holds true: You cannot get grant funding if you do not submit an application. Even if the odds are low for funding, it is important to try, as a nurse investigator or team never knows up front how grant funders and grant reviewers will view the project. It may be the only submittal that showcases research that is novel, important, and meaningful in relation to current political, environmental, or clinical events.

The details required on grant applications can be mystifying to novice researchers, and development of the application, proposal, budget, and bio sketch are time consuming. Doctorate-prepared nurse researchers with a strong background in grant writing and funding will be able to provide the necessary support for successful grant applications.

There are many Internet sites and books available that provide steps to grant writing and receiving grant support. In two novel programs, multiple small hospitals can join into a multisite study by providing funding for project initiation and ongoing overhead costs, such as proposal writing and orientation of sites, database development, analysis of data, and dissemination back to sites (Hickey, Koithan, Unruh, & Lundmark, 2014; Improvement Science Research Network [isrn.net]). An important element of funding is that a well-written and impactful grant is of primary importance; it should clearly and concisely describe the potential benefits of the research to multiprofessional groups. Funders want to believe that their money is well spent. Funders will assess the research team for follow through by reviewing previous publication efforts. Curriculum vitae that reflect a solid publication history and previous funding will be important assets. The novice clinical nurse, however, may not have a history of publication and funding. To overcome a weak curriculum vita in regard to research, it is very important to include research mentors as co-investigators who have research doctorate credentials, a history of grant support, an escalating publication history in peer-reviewed journals, and expertise that is specific to one or more aspects of the research topic. Since part of the research process includes statistical analysis, always include a biostatistician as a co-investigator. Additionally, include multiprofessional experts as collaborators and mentors, and provide letters of support from the principal investigator's supervisor and expert consultants when allowed. Table 7.1 contains a summary of some helpful tips to getting grant funding.

Academic–Clinical Partnership: Graduate Degree *Student Research Practicum*

Nurses working on graduate degrees often need to receive practical nursing research experiences as a requirement toward graduation. Nursing research practicum requirements expose nurses to research processes and related work that may stimulate an interest in leading research. More important to the nursing research program, graduate level research practica provide an important resource: service, which equates to time. Hours of practica experiences completed by students decrease the requirement of time needed by principal and co-investigators. The nursing department and hospital organization can also use the hours spent in supporting collegiate clinical research practica as part of community service.

When giving time toward educating students in research and providing administrative oversight to ensure work is accurately based on good clinical research practice expectations, nurse researcher leaders must consider costs to the nursing research department. The biggest cost is time, but needed resources may also include physical space, computer and telephone access, and lab costs. An assessment of the benefits of participating in student research practicums to the nursing research program and nursing department will ensure the program is advantageous and does not drain precious resources that should be devoted to hospital personnel rather than students.

TABLE 7.1 Grant Funding Tips

THEME	TIPS
Understanding the requirements of the grant	• Begin early (4 months or more ahead of the application deadline for the grant) to review grant application requirements and begin writing your proposal. • Carefully read and follow every detail of the information in the grant application. • Call the contact person noted in the grant application with any questions to clarify any requirements. • If you are not able to meet *every* requirement for the grant application, move on to another grant.
Writing the grant proposal	• Obtain help and mentorship from someone who has already written a grant proposal (preferably successfully) similar to the one you are considering. • Begin writing very early and dedicate regular time to work on it. • Be sure to describe the potential positive impact of your findings throughout the proposal. • Do not get creative; format your proposal *exactly* as the grant application requires. • Have colleagues and mentors review your proposal for grammar, spelling, and clarity.
Put together a strong research team	• If you, the principal investigator, are not yet well-published, include a co-investigator with a strong history of published work in the area of interest. • Include another expert as co-investigator if necessary to support your ability to complete the research if the grant is awarded. • Include a bio-statistician if possible to support your ability to accurately analyze data and disseminate findings.
Proof of additional support	• Obtain letters of support from administrators and others who are directly in a position to support your research, data collection, and dissemination of findings. • List infrastructure support, adequate population to collect your sample without difficulty, and other resources that will make your research feasible.
Get information for new grant opportunities	• Make lists of professional organizations that provide grant funding and keep up with their funding websites. • Sign up for regular e-mails on funding opportunities through the National Institutes of Health (NIH) grants.nih.gov/grants/guide/listserv.htm.
Innovative ideas for professional guidance and funding	• Consider participating in pay-to-participate funding through organizations such as the American Nurses Credentialing Center (ANCC). • Consider crowd-source funding through professional organizations (Hickey et al., 2014).

Academic–Clinical Partnership: Graduate Degree Program *Intensive Course*

Many nursing graduate degree programs include a clinical course near the end of the program that focuses on leadership in a patient population, or in education, administration, or informatics. Receiving an intensive experience with a leader of a nursing research program can be beneficial to students through growth in a research context, and also to the nursing research department, through the hours of student services provided. The latter is especially true if students assist with nursing research structure development as part of the experience. For example, in an intensive course students may assist with creating new templates, checklists, or step-by-step handouts on a research theme; complete a literature review and synthesis of evidence on a topic of interest to the program; or develop a novel way to enhance nurses' use of evidence-based practice resources. This type of clinical does not focus on allowing students to assist with individual research projects; rather, it gives time toward meeting a program need, filling a gap, or expanding services and resources.

Nursing research program leaders need to develop relationships with graduate program deans to increase their awareness of support for students completing an intensive course in nursing research. Similar to students completing research practica, exposure to clinical nursing research programs may create a passion and excitement for research and high-quality evidence-based practices that may endure and be enhanced after graduation.

RESEARCH EDUCATION FOR NURSES

Nursing research education and resources are essential to the success of a high-quality, rigorous nursing research program. Although there is a growing understanding that utilization of evidence-based practice and implementation of research are important to the professional development of nurses, nurses may be unsure about how to start a research project, or how to overcome barriers once they get a nursing research project started. Without adequate knowledge of research processes, novice nurse researchers may initiate a project that is poor quality or has multiple internal and external threats to validity. Poorly designed and executed research minimizes the study's contribution to the science of nursing. Clinical research can be complex, even for highly motivated clinicians, and requires extra education and guidance from research experts. When expert nurse researchers share their own program of research findings, especially lessons learned in hindsight, it may stimulate nurses to consider gaps, issues, problems and new ideas that require further study.

Meeting Primary Research Education Needs

A major barrier to getting nursing research started and ongoing research completed is a lack of knowledge of research processes and a lack of experts who can provide education that is specific to the needs of individual research projects. Hospital-based nurse educators and administrators may not have sufficient knowledge themselves regarding the important role of nursing research and an understanding of how to complete high-quality nursing research studies (Tanner & Hale, 2002). To get interested nurses started on the path to research, basic research education must be easily accessible.

VOICES OF NURSE RESEARCHERS

Connie White-Williams, PhD, RN, FAAN
Director, Center for Nursing Excellence, Assistant Professor,
School of Nursing, University of Alabama at Birmingham Hospital,
Birmingham, Alabama

Most nurses that I mentor have a question or a curiosity that they want to explore. Nurses who are in school work with their schools of nursing and usually do not use hospital resources. Time is the biggest barrier, and I encourage nurses to have a conversation with their nurse manager before beginning a research project. At our hospital, nurses know to contact the Center for Nursing Excellence (CNE) and the CNE staff will help them with their research, evidence-based practice (EBP), or quality projects. We are fortunate that the departments of Quality, Research, EBP, and Education originate from the CNE. We work as a team to assist nursing staff.

Finding a way to incorporate research into other programs has been successful for our hospital. We require all nurses in the clinical ladder program to become IRB trained. This requirement provides the necessary education for nurses to engage in research studies. We offer workshops on nursing research, how to complete an IRB application, how to search the literature, abstract development, oral and poster presentations, and writing for publication. We also provide mentorship to assist nurses through the research process. These resources come from the CNE.

Cynthia Bautista, PhD, RN, CNRN, SCRN, CCNS, ACNS-BC, FNCS
Neuroscience Clinical Nurse Specialist, Yale–New Haven Hospital,
New Haven, Connecticut

I have assisted many staff nurses who wanted to do a research study and did not know where to turn. I enjoy sitting with staff nurses to discuss their ideas about clinical problems. I like to use the Iowa Model of Evidence-Based Practice (Titler et al., 2001) and, in 10 easy steps, assist staff nurses to create clinical questions, search for evidence, and determine if research studies are needed or if there is enough evidence to make practice changes.

Basic Research Education and Resources

Basic research knowledge should be available and conveniently accessible to individuals, no matter their work schedules. It must also have a format that allows for self-paced learning. Some examples include library access to research tutorials, scientific journals, and professional organizations' evidence-based practice databases. Easily-accessible online research education and resources can fill an education gap, and if self-assessment is included, nurses may better understand their current level of knowledge and future educational needs. As online education matures and becomes more interactive, nurses may be more willing to use it. For example, many colleges now offer massive open online courses (MOOCs) in nursing research. Locally, nurse researchers can encourage MOOC participation and offer in-person education and knowledge that supplements MOOC content through weekly or monthly question-and-answer sessions or other formats.

Additionally, nurses should be able to browse and retrieve research from website resources. For example, nurse researchers may provide multiple listings of validated and reliable instruments on common outcomes (e.g., patient pain, anxiety, and depression, or nurse satisfaction, retention, and burnout) used by nurses in research. Other resources include providing research templates and posters of completed research by nursing peers. Chapter 3 discusses specific research templates and other resources that can serve to educate nurses who are novices in research.

Research Workshops

Basic or advanced nursing research workshops that are interactive and include demonstration may encourage or inspire nurses to advance in nursing research. Workshops can vary in overall length and in the percentage of time devoted to practice and group discussions. Some examples are:

- Getting started in research
- How to conduct a literature review
- How to develop a database
- How to develop a theoretical or conceptual model
- Proposal writing 101
- Designing a randomized controlled trial
- Fun with statistics

In a proposal-writing workshop, small groups can practice writing a pretend proposal. Then they can share and discuss their work with all attendees. Pretend proposals may turn into actual, rigorous, and valuable nursing research.

Unit-Based Research Education

Research education and incentives may need to be worked into the flow of nurses' work shifts. Thirty-minute staff meetings or lunch-and-learn presentations on specific research themes and even on available resources can spark research interest. As a follow-up to brief meetings/presentations, nurses may need electronic or paper go-to resources and researcher contact information. To enhance research education on nursing units, posters were created on *Internet Resources in Nursing Research*; *Quality Improvement Versus Quality Research*; *Steps of the Research Process*; and *Translating Research Knowledge into Clinical Practice*. The four themes were selected as they are universally applicable, no matter the clinical setting. Nurse managers can print poster content on 11 × 17 inch paper and post in unit lounges.

Annual Nursing Research Conference

One fun way of exposing clinical nurses to nurse-led research and providing basic and advanced research education is to hold a nursing research conference. Keynote speakers can be leaders in nursing research (locally or nationally known) who share their program of research and findings, or those who provide a review of key themes of importance to the hospital organization or nursing department. Even if messages received are similar to messages delivered previously by local leaders, when external experts deliver content, nurses may be more likely to take next steps. A research conference promotes networking among colleagues, provides new views on current problems, encourages collaboration with other nurse researchers, and may stimulate new research questions. The chief nursing officer should be invited to provide opening remarks or a welcome address. In that way, clinical nurses will hear leadership support for nursing research and better understand why it is essential to nursing's mission. Including a call for research abstracts for oral and poster presentations will provide practical knowledge to novice nurse researchers and allow them to share their research findings.

CONCLUSION

Since contributions of nursing research are vital to the science and art of nursing and provide the foundation for evidence-based practices, it is important to overcome the traditional cluster of barriers that include problems with nursing research visibility/priority, time and money, and research education. Nurses need confirmation that nurse leaders support research; when it is visible, it is valued. Moreover, nurses need time, education, and resources to complete rigorous research that leads to discoveries and answers to important clinical problems.

REFERENCES

American Nurses Association. (2010). *Nursing's Social Policy Statement: The Essence of the Profession*. Silver Spring, MD: Author.

Aiello-Laws, L. B., Clark, J., Steele-Moses, S., Jardine, S., & McGee, L. (2010). Oncology Nursing Society Journal Club How-to Guide. Retrieved May 10, 2011 from http://www.ons.org

Chulay, M. (2006). Good research ideas for clinicians. *AACN Advanced Critical Care*, 17, 253–265.

Cleveland Clinic. (2014). Career development. Retrieved November 7, 2014 from http://my.clevelandclinic.org/services/nursing-institute/career-growth-development/career-development

Donley, R., & Flaherty, R. (2008). Promoting professional development: Three phases of articulation in nursing education and practice. *The Online Journal of Issues in Nursing*. Retrieved from http://www.nursingworld.org/MainMenuCategories/ANAMarketplace/ANAPeriodicals/OJIN/TableofContents/vol132008/No3Sept08/PhasesofArticulation.aspx

Duke Nursing. (2014). Clinical ladder. Retrieved November 7, 2014 from http://www.dukenursing.org/programs/clinical-ladder/

Hickey, J. V., Koithan, M., Unruh, L., & Lundmark, V. (2014). Funding big research with small money. *Journal of Nursing Administration*, 44(6), 309–312.

LoBiondo-Wood, G., & Haber, J. (Eds.). (2013). *Nursing research: Methods and critical appraisal for evidence-based practice*. St. Louis, MO: Elsevier Health Sciences.

Penn State Hershey. (2014). Clinical ladder. Retrieved November 7, 2014 from: http://www.pennstatehershey.org/web/nursing/home/overview/professionaldevelopment/clinicalladder

Saladino, L., & Gosselin, T. (2014). Budgeting nursing time to support unit-based clinical inquiry. *AACN Advanced Critical Care*, 25(3), 291–296.

Tanner, J., & Hale, C. (2002). Research-active nurses' perceptions of the barriers to undertaking research in practice. *Nursing Times Research*, 7(5), 363–375.

Titler, M. G., Kleiber, C., Steelman, V. J., Rakel, B. A., Budreau, G., Everett, L. Q., . . . Goode, C. J. (2001). The Iowa Model of evidence-based practice to promote quality care. *Critical Care Nursing Clinics of North America*, 13, 497–509.

Westlake, C., Albert, N. M., Rice, K. L., Bautista, C., Close, J., Foster, J., & Timmerman, G. M. (2015). Nursing journal clubs and the clinical nurse specialist. *Clinical Nurse Specialist*, 29(1): E1–E10. doi: 10.1097/NUR.0000000000000095

Nancy M. Albert
Roberta Cwynar
Donna M. Ross

8

TRANSLATING RESEARCH INTO CLINICAL PRACTICE

This chapter focuses on translating nursing research into practice. No matter if the clinical research intervention to be implemented into practice was designed, developed, and implemented in the same hospital where the translation will occur, or if new knowledge came from a published research paper, usually the translation phase is the hardest part of research work. Creating and maintaining a culture of evidence-based practice (EBP; see Chapter 1) is essential to fostering translation of new knowledge into practice. To aid new researchers in considering the many elements of translation that need to happen, we developed an algorithm (Figure 8.1).

Since translation of research into practice may not always be successful, some researchers set out to determine factors that might be most important. When assessing interventions that led to success in 27 U.S. Agency for Healthcare Research and Quality (AHRQ)-funded applications that were intended to prompt translation of research, the most common interventions used were adult learning theory and organizational theory. Also, more than half of the projects used information technology (Farquhar, Stryer, & Slutsky, 2002). Although theories that promote education and organizational behaviors are important, in hospital units where clinical nurses complete shift work, other factors may need to be considered to translate new knowledge into practice.

Historically, there has been a time lag in health care research translation processes. In a review of 23 papers, the mean lag time was 17 years and authors commented that the literature on this topic was underdeveloped, especially since some lag time was due to publication delays by authors. Other reasons for lags in health care research translation were publication bias (failure to publish null or negative reports and speed of publication by journal publishers—publishing positive outcomes more quickly than negative

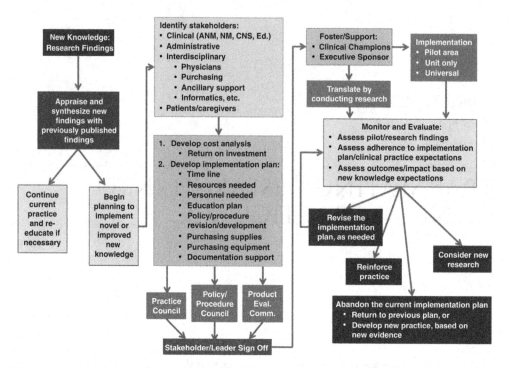

FIGURE 8.1 Cleveland Clinic Nursing Institute Translation of New Knowledge Into Practice.
Source: The Office of Nursing Research and Innovation, Cleveland Clinic (2015).

outcomes) and research domain; for example, time to support clinical use of thrombolytic drugs after a myocardial infarction was short (6 years), whereas parenteral nutrition took 21 years (Morris, Wooding & Grant, 2011).

When researchers assessed translation of guidelines into clinical practice, there were many factors that affected it (Davis & Taylor-Vaisey, 1997). Of the characteristics of health care professionals, younger age of medical graduates was associated with higher likelihood of following guidelines. Of characteristics of practice settings, system efficiencies (e.g., plans to discharge patients on weekends, when applicable) and implementation plans that overcame issues were factors. Incentives and federal and other regulations also prompted translation (Davis & Taylor-Vaisey, 1997). Researchers adapted a cascade of steps needed to influence adoption of guidelines. Practitioner knowledge, skills, attitudes, and behaviors all influenced clinical experiences and implementation, and led to patient or health care outcomes that also affected clinical experiences and implantation (Davis & Taylor-Vaisey, 1997). Based on these findings, health care providers' willingness to adapt to change and adopt new knowledge and practices can make a difference in successful translation of research.

To speed adoption of research into practice, it is important to consider lessons learned by others. Bradley et al. (2004) listed the following seven lessons that were key to translation:

- Senior management and effective clinical leadership support
- Credible data that can persuade administrators who make budget decisions
- Implementation plan that does not require heavy organizational culture changes
- Less need to coordinate implementation plans across departments or disciplines
- Infrastructure that includes personnel with expertise and needed resources
- A dissemination infrastructure that more closely matches the adopting organization (can be mutual commitment to the intervention or a contract that binds the two entities)
- Perceptions that research implementation will reduce external threats

Of these seven lessons, all are directly or indirectly included in Figure 8.1, including reducing external threats. For some interventions, external threats may feel remote, and may require key stakeholders to think beyond day-to-day practice. For example, if the intervention is aimed at improving a quality metric (falls, infection, or pressure ulcers) on one nursing unit, it may be important for key stakeholders to consider the influence of improved quality outcomes on Centers for Medicare & Medicaid Services, National Quality Forum, and The Joint Commission requirements.

In the next three sections of this chapter, elements of the algorithm are described based on what is known in the literature. The algorithm begins with considerations after research findings are finalized. Decisions made in this early phase are based on a review of the literature. For novice researchers, a mentor or coach may aid in synthesizing new findings with contemporary literature. In the second section, the focus is on taking the steps needed to bring the research intervention to life. As shown in Figure 8.1, there are multiple considerations that involve both people and processes. The focus in the third section is on two building blocks: (a) translation by implementing the intervention or (b) translation by conducting research and assessment of outcomes. Both elements are needed to determine sustainability of the translated intervention.

EARLY TRANSLATION WORK

A personal desire to bring a research intervention to daily practice and researcher authority in implementing an intervention may not be enough to overcome the complicated processes of research translation. Multiple processes and factors must align (similar to making the right interconnections of a puzzle piece for all four sides). The first step is to determine how new findings relate to previous research findings.

Appraise and Synthesize New Findings With Previously Published Findings

The findings of new research need to be evaluated in relation to the intervention. Questions to ask are: Should the new intervention (practice or improvement) be implemented? What is the effect of the new practice in improving outcomes? Are real world subjects similar to the research population? Can the research effect be expected to have similar results when the intervention is applied in the same population of real-world subjects (or more globally)? Besides the expected effects, will a practice change affect subjects in other, nonstudied ways? Will there be a return on investment, and if so, when is it likely to be felt? Consider the effects of implementing an intervention on staff or patient satisfaction. Think about costs (associated with implementation and maintenance of the intervention) or other factors that may be altered by the intervention.

Of all questions, the most important to answer is: Why should we translate new findings? The Robert Wood Johnson Foundation and Institute for Healthcare Improvement *Transforming Care at the Bedside* program was carried out over a 5-year period (2003–2008) to engage clinical caregivers as local leaders of change and improvement efforts. Many researchers found benefits, such as improved quality of health care, patient safety, and caregiver efficiencies, as well as enhanced teamwork and reduced costs of care (Dearmon et al., 2013; Unruh, Agrawal, & Hassmiller, 2011). Equally important to asking why it is important to translate new knowledge, it is also important to consider untold effects of implementing a new intervention, practice, or improvement. For some interventions, there may be many indirect benefits or harms that are not discovered until after the intervention becomes more widely used in a real-world setting. A literature review may reveal new knowledge that was not available when the research was begun. A literature review and synthesis of findings may strengthen or weaken your desire to make a clinical change in practice. Review of current literature will offer critical information to assist with decisions about moving forward and help in the development of the implementation plan. It is necessary to review what others found concerning the new knowledge and develop a consensus regarding taking action. Ultimately, a synthesis of the literature will strengthen your ability to explain why the intervention should be adopted. Reference data might also help build a plan that addresses concerns that might be raised during implementation discussions.

Appraising and synthesizing new findings with previously published findings is often difficult because many health care providers do not understand how to complete a scoping (systematic) review of the literature on a theme/topic and need managerial support for education time with a coach before decisions about next steps can be made. In a systematic review that involved both doctors and nurses, attitudes toward EBPs were positive, but major stumbling blocks were: (a) knowledge of EBP terms (such as odds ratio, funnel plot, relative odds ratio reduction, heterogeneity, weighted mean difference, and others) that affect understanding of study findings, and (b) making ideal decisions regarding study implications (readiness for translation into clinical practice; Ubbink, Guyatt, & Vermeulen, 2013). Core literature may be difficult to assess, either because it is scattered among many diverse books and journals, or because it is overwhelming in size/scope. Not only are empirical studies needed (or systematic reviews of empirical studies on the theme/topic), but the review of literature may also include relevant theoretical constructs and methodological issues (Rubenstein & Pugh, 2006).

Even when research and related evidence is clear and understandable, it is not always clear what organizational intervention steps enhance adoption of best practice. In papers reviewed as part of a systematic review of decision making by clinicians, three organizational elements were used to advance adoption of best practice: a knowledge broker, access to systematic reviews, and provision of tailored messages; yet there were no differences in program planning among groups with and without these elements (Murthy et al., 2012). In other reports included in the systematic review, printed bulletins of evidence from systematic reviews on a specific treatment/intervention were effective in prompting clinicians to make practice changes (Murthy et al., 2012). Thus, using a printed bulletin with a single clear message that summarizes systematic review evidence may improve awareness of EBP.

Ultimately, if the intention is to develop awareness and knowledge of a review of evidence on an intervention that is part of new knowledge, nurses must have skills in interpreting evidence and also in developing a multifaceted intervention that addresses best practice needs. Proposed solutions may include organizational level interventions such as using national and international associations and hospital management to promote EBP, education, and individual support through clinical unit leaders who can guide teams in moving evidence from the discussion page of a research paper to the bedside.

Continue Current Practice and Reeducate if Necessary

When new research findings support current standards of practice, it is important to reassess actual practices to determine the level of synchrony between policies and procedures and actual behaviors. If there is a match between current practice and intervention expectations, a discussion about ongoing continuation, maintenance needs, and actions needed to foster persistence may strengthen support of current practices and promote refinements that promote sustainability. In one report, a panel of experts suggested that health program sustainability required context and resources related to positive and negative drivers of the intervention and interactions between the health concerns that prompted intervention implementation, research (or quality) results, and political economy (that considers how key stakeholders influence the intervention, barriers, or shortfalls to achieving success and level of engagement in supporting the intervention; Gruen et al., 2008).

When there is a mismatch between documented highest evidence/best practice and actual behaviors, communication and education of new research may reinforce standards of practice and provide rationale for current best practices behaviors. Staff education may foster discussions that raise awareness of an intervention's importance, and may promote systematic implementation (same time, place, and/or expected actions) and documentation of behaviors. Finally, re-education reinforces why nurses act the way they do and serves as a reminder that research should support practice. When workplace effectiveness is not in line with standards of practice, nurses may state that they do not have enough time (Clark & Thompson, 2014). Time is a resource that can be mapped to priorities and used based on personal decisions (choice), but it is not amenable to management in the same way as processes of care are. Nurses must choose and allocate time toward the right priorities and understand how to ignore or minimize time spent on nonpriorities (Clark & Thompson, 2014). Education of current practice expectations in a way that creates value and meaning for the expected behavior itself and of subsequent outcomes might help overcome issues that are rooted in time and prioritization.

Begin Planning to Implement Novel or Improved New Knowledge

When research is completed and a decision is made to implement new or improved knowledge or interventions, planning (or strategizing) is needed. A narrative culture, in which clinical narratives become part of the fabric of professional life, may aid in the process (Benner, 1984), but there may still be organizational barriers related to workplace setting, administrative support, and infrastructure resources. Further, patient preferences and clinician expertise should be part of decision making. When intervention implementation decisions are not clearly obvious, the implementation plan may involve pilot, efficacy, and effectiveness testing before diffusion toward widespread adoption.

BRINGING RESEARCH TRANSLATION TO LIFE

There are many translation models available in the literature. Some focus on the steps or phases of movement from discovery to implementation in practice and use time and processes as markers of forward movement. For example, in one model, authors use five phases to show research movement. The first phase is research involving scientific discovery (Time 0). Subsequent phases are movement to candidate application (Time 1), to evidence-based recommendation or policy (Time 2), to practice and control programs (Time 3) and finally, to population health impact (Time 4; Khoury, Gwinn & Ioannidis, 2010). The AHRQ knowledge transfer framework (Nieva et al., 2005) uses three distinct processes—(a) knowledge creation and distillation; (b) diffusion and dissemination; and (c) adoption, implementation, and institutionalization—to show forward movement toward distillation of research in clinical practice. The framework provides target audiences and activities for each of the three process phases.

Models that are the most applicable to translating hospital-based nursing research into practice are those that consider more than just phases and processes of translation. It is important for nurses to understand the context in which translation of research into practice occurs by understanding the structures and processes involved in adoption of innovation. Rogers's Diffusion of Innovations Theory provides a framework for implementing research into practice. Rogers's framework includes four elements (in italics)—an *innovation* is *communicated* or shared to reach mutual understanding over *time*, among members of a *social system* (Rogers, 2003). The social system involves structure, norms, opinion leadership, and change agents that are all interrelated and can influence a decision to adopt innovation. In Rogers's theory, an innovation will take off and have greater chances for success when the rate of adoption to use the innovation as a best course of action is at least 20%. Earlier adoption and a fast takeoff above 20% use will aid success; however, the rate of adoption can be slowed (or even terminated) when the perceived attributes of the innovation are not well understood, when communication channels are unclear, when norms and other elements of the social system are not interconnected, and when change agents do not promote the innovation adequately (Rogers, 2003). Rogers's Diffusion of Innovations Theory provides realistic considerations for changing clinician behavior and has been applied in promoting diabetes self-management, for example (Titler, 2007).

The AHRQ developed a Translating Research into Practice (TRIP)-I initiative to overcome translation hurdles that were ongoing despite reminder systems, local opinion leaders, computer decision support systems, and financial incentives aimed at implementing research into practice (AHRQ, 2001). Government leaders recognized that it could take up to two decades for original, pragmatic research to be implemented in daily clinical practice. In TRIP-I, researchers carried out translational research to promote the use of rigorous new knowledge in practice. In TRIP-I, translation methods were carried out in idealized practice settings. In TRIP-II, the focus turned to applying and assessing strategies developed in TRIP-I in diverse clinical settings. TRIP-II projects involved collaborative partnerships and use of information technology to promote success (AHRQ, 2001), both of which are consistent with Rogers's diffusion theory in regard to communication and social systems. However, effectiveness of translation strategies that focused on consumers of health care were not always effective (Grimshaw, Eccles, Lavis, Hill, & Squire, 2012). For example, in systematic reviews, decision aids were effective in improving knowledge and reducing passivity in decision making, written information resulted in mixed outcomes, self-management programs had short-term improvements, and personalized risk communication, communication before consultations, and some interventions with new methods of communicating all failed to meet outcome expectations due to little or no effect on behaviors (Grimshaw et al., 2012). Ultimately, Grimshaw et al. (2012) recommend answering five questions:

- What new research knowledge should be transferred?
- To whom should research knowledge be transferred?
- By whom should research knowledge be transferred?
- How should research knowledge be transferred?
- With what effect should research knowledge be transferred?

Answers to these five questions will be based on themes discussed in the next section.

Identifying Stakeholders

Identifying all stakeholders involved in translation of research into practice is essential. An assessment of stakeholders' readiness for practice change and consideration of how practice change may affect each stakeholder should be considered. Depending on the answer to "To whom should knowledge be transferred?," hospital stakeholders may vary, but generally include administration, nursing leadership, clinical experts, physicians, nursing educators, purchasing, ancillary departments, information technology, patients, and patients' supporters/caregivers. Other stakeholders may include national specialty organizations and government officials.

Administrative support within the organization is essential for translation of new knowledge into practice. Lack of administration support and administrative leaders who do not model EBP were identified as barriers to translating new evidence-based interventions into practice (Melnyk & Morrison-Beedy, 2012). In one report, Bradley and colleagues conducted case studies on four empirically proven effective innovative clinical programs. The first lesson learned was that strong support of senior management at the adopting organization increased the success of adoption (Bradley et al., 2004).

External factors such as federal health policies, regulations, and reimbursement policies can influence administrative support for implementing new knowledge into practice. In an era of value-based purchasing and limited resources, administration may be more willing to support and provide resources to implement new knowledge into practice if improved patient outcomes are demonstrated and supported in the literature. For example, interventions that decrease ventilator-associated pneumonia, central line blood stream infections, catheter-associated urinary tract infections, and 30-day hospital readmissions or interventions with a strong effect on improving patient satisfaction scores may have a higher priority and increased support because financial penalties are assessed.

Support from clinical management teams is an essential facilitator of or barrier to implementing new knowledge into practice. When considering "How should research knowledge be transferred?," not only should environmental, financial, and political facilitators and barriers be considered to inform the choice of translation strategy, but nurse managers, assistant nurse managers, clinical nurse specialists, and nurse educators are key drivers of organizational change. Nursing leaders must understand the value of the practice change and be committed to it for adoption and diffusion to be successful. Nursing cultures that do not support EBP and organizations that lack EBP mentors have been identified as barriers to translating evidence-based innovations into clinical practice (Melnyk & Morrison-Beedy, 2012). Furthermore, effective clinical leadership speeds adoption of new practice in an organization (Bradley et al., 2004).

To be successful implementing new knowledge into practice, support and commitment from interdisciplinary personnel must be considered. Physicians, pharmacy, informatics, purchasing, and other ancillary support within the organization may be resistant to implementing new findings because they perceive the change as having little value to improved outcomes. In some cases, interdisciplinary providers may have invested capital in an alternative approach that they are unwilling to abandon, there may be financial disincentives to adopting new practices, or there may be current or future budget constraints and higher perceived priorities. Building a cohesive interdisciplinary team where all the members perceive the practice change as valuable to patient outcome and to the organization is crucial. Implementing the new practices or processes slows when the change requires coordination and collaboration among disciplines and across departments (Bradley et al., 2004).

Patients and their support teams should be the primary stakeholders considered when decisions are made about implementing clinical practice changes aimed at quality patient outcomes. At the Cleveland Clinic, we use the phrase "patients first" to reflect our focus on delivery of high-quality patient care, every time. Our phrase is reminiscent of a statement by an AHRQ leader, who felt that quality care within organizations and health care delivery systems was more than the right people and facilities. Rather, quality was determined by ensuring patients received the right decisions and care in the right way (What is Health Care Quality and Who Decides?, 2009). When resistance to changing practice occurs from providers and among department administrators, it is important to build a case for change by disseminating supportive data that show improved patient outcomes and demonstrating the necessity of improving quality of care as a key driver to changing practice.

Developing a Cost Analysis

An important step required for translating new knowledge into practice is to perform a cost analysis. It is important to determine if the cost of implementing and evaluating the practice change yields a return on investment. Factors that need to be calculated into the cost analysis include all resources needed for educating, implementing, evaluating, and sustaining the new practice. Cost of productive time for all personnel, in all departments, and among all providers needs to be taken into account. Cost for supplies and equipment, developing policy and procedures, documentation support, and data abstraction need to be calculated into the overall cost. If new knowledge only provides a minimal change in clinical outcomes (limited/small effect size), it may not be prudent to invest valuable, limited resources on a practice change.

When determining total costs of supplies and equipment, there are several considerations beyond direct costs. Labor (time) cost for evaluating products and associated equipment, negotiating pricing of supplies, equipment, and purchasing contracts, and labor associated with maintaining, cleaning, and disposing of products are important indirect costs. Further, education and communication that may need to be ongoing for a period of time add to costs of practice changes. Instructor class time and time to prepare education content/plan, continuing education credits, and materials must be included as costs in addition to participant time away from clinical nursing work. Labor costs also include nurse educators needed for round-the-clock in-servicing and electronic mail correspondence related to education and competency. If an online learning module is created, time (in hours) needed to develop and proofread the learning module and to make revisions based on a set schedule (yearly) need to be considered. Ongoing informatics technical support is often required to ensure smooth operability when accessed, and for making changes as new knowledge emerges or when there are computer or programming glitches.

Major revisions of policy can be costly, since it may be labor intensive, especially when more than one department is involved in the practice change, and it involves review by multiple stakeholders. Members of the policy committee need time to evaluate the literature, discuss the practice change, determine how the change will affect multidisciplinary processes, and come to a consensus on new policies or procedures. If several revisions are needed before the final policy is completed, and if several committees must sign off before implementation, labor costs may mount.

Documentation and data collection (quality improvement) costs need to be included in a cost analysis. Labor costs to design or change documentation in electronic medical records can be steep and may involve outside contracts with the established informatics vendor. When created internally, product evaluation of documentation changes may take time and add to costs, especially if multiple solutions are needed before the system is finalized. Moreover, additional labor cost to abstract data manually or via electronic data pull for performance improvement or outcomes assessment must be calculated into the cost analysis.

Developing an Implementation Plan

Nurses cannot be left to "just do it" when it comes to developing an implementation plan. Clinicians may be cognitively aware of new knowledge from explicit declarative information presented to them, but cognitive processes are needed to shift (or translate) declarative information in action. An "if–then" framework may help make the process of developing an implementation plan easier (Green & Seifert, 2005). "If" consists of the conditions needed to apply new knowledge based on understanding of the facts, and "then" reflects the specific actions to be taken. An "if–then" framework creates procedural rules that can be followed in clinical settings.

Creating a timeline is an important step, as it facilitates an organized process for the implementation of the new practice. Setting realistic goals for specific tasks that need to be completed before implementation of practice changes decreases stress and gives all stakeholders, including external vendors, a global perspective of work criteria and deadlines. The practice-change leader can also use the timeline to communicate expected and actual milestones and quality/performance achievements.

It is important to assess all resources needed and personnel involved in the process of changing practice. Systems and personnel barriers to practice change need to be removed when possible, and incentives for change need to be understood and facilitated. A careful assessment of the number of EBP mentors within the organization and EBP expert champions at the unit level helps to determine overall support. More direct and indirect support may lead to early success in implementing and sustaining new research findings into practice. Nurses who were viewed by their peers as respectful and competent are informal leaders of behavior change and can influence group norms (Titler, 2007). In one report, opinion leaders—defined as people from the local peer group who were thought of as technically competent and a respected source of influence—who utilized EBP and supported practice change influenced peers' perceptions of the value of the practice change and influenced behavior to adopt change (Titler, 2007).

The implementation plan must include a detailed education plan. The number of nurse educators available, the number of people who need to be educated, and the education delivery methods will influence how the education plan is developed and carried out. An important consideration is the match between education delivery strategies and learning objectives needed to implement the new practice. Can the education be provided through an online learning course, or is it important to have in-person classroom discussions or nursing unit demonstrations and return demonstrations by the learner? Is a posttest sufficient to evaluate mastery of content or is visual evaluation of competency required? The types and complexity of education needed will affect the time commitments required of staff and learners to ensure competency. Before education can begin, policy and procedure development or revisions need to be completed. Educating on a new practice without making changes in the policy will lead to confusion and practice inconsistencies. Further, if the practice change requires new or altered documentation in the electronic medical record, testing should be completed before education is started.

A well-developed implementation plan will account for the availability of supplies and equipment. Can the practice change be implemented with current supplies and equipment or does it require new or altered supplies and equipment? Delays will occur if new supplies and medical equipment need to be purchased, assessed after delivery, stocked on units, and/or evaluated for quality. Market pricing and availability of products need to be considered in the implementation plan.

At the Cleveland Clinic, the implementation plan is evaluated by three main shared-governance councils (Practice Council, Policy and Procedure Council, and Product Evaluation Committee) and approved by leadership. The Practice Council consists of nursing leaders and advanced practice nurses who represent all hospital organizations within the Cleveland Clinic Health System. Council representatives evaluate the evidence, decide if implementation is feasible, identify safety concerns, and discuss important findings that shape nursing practice. The Policy and Procedure Committee develops policy using wording that applies to all hospital organization sites. To facilitate policy approval without multiple revisions, committee members consider the variability in internal factors at each site, such as the type of personnel on units, number of unit-based experts, computer technology and equipment needs at each site, and financial resources. For example, nurse call systems, bed features, and nurse-to-nurse communication may differ by nursing unit, based on upgrade schedules and original equipment. A practice change that involves bed alarm features may need to be very global to meet the needs of all participating units. The Cleveland Clinic Nursing Institute model for translation of new knowledge into practice encourages multidisciplinary stakeholders to evaluate research findings and develop and implement practice based on high-quality evidence. Once the Practice Council, Policy and Procedure Council, and Product Evaluation Committee come to consensus on best practice and approve a policy, it is signed off by the main stakeholders, nursing leaders, and the board of governors.

Fostering Support

To achieve successful implementation of practice changes, both clinical champions and an executive sponsor are needed to aid in optimizing communication within and among team members and to foster networking, as needed. Local peers should be recruited to be champions of implementing research interventions. Clinical champions should be informal leaders; that is, non-managerial people who are respected by staff. Clinical champions need to be educated on the practice change so they can discuss and reinforce the steps of the intervention and provide rationale for initiating the practice change. Once the practice change is initiated, clinical champions can be the eyes and ears of staff members in terms of auditing the implementation to ensure it is realistic and to provide feedback that will contribute to successful implementation of the practice change.

As discussed previously in identifying stakeholders, senior leadership support is needed prior to implementing new research findings. Senior leadership should demonstrate active engagement and a willingness to show support for the practice change within leadership working groups and more globally (e.g., via newsletter and intranet messages, by recognizing the group for their efforts, and by asking stakeholders and clinical champions to present implementation outcomes to leadership personnel). Senior leadership support may be also viewed as release time for teams to finalize and implement the practice change. Senior leadership support is crucial to assisting in practice change sustainability over time, especially if costs need to be defrayed and external threats need to be overcome.

TRANSLATION THROUGH IMPLEMENTATION OF PRACTICE CHANGES AND NEW RESEARCH

Implementation of Practice Changes

Implementation of research into practice proceeds through three stages: awareness of new knowledge, acceptance of new knowledge as best practice and highest quality evidence, and, finally, implementation in practice (Green & Seifert, 2005). Implementation of new knowledge into practice may be carried out on a small scale; for example, on one nursing unit as a pilot project or more globally. The decision to go small or large in implementing practice changes may be based on many of the factors previously discussed: the number of potential barriers and facilitators to practice changes identified, level of stakeholder support and encouragement, level of purchased resources needed to successfully implement change, degree of disruption in services expected by the practice change, availability of the appropriate staff to implement change, complexity and multifaceted nature of the intervention or practice change, complexity of education needed, level and complexity of communication and decision making involved in the practice change, and resources needed to assess performance/quality of outcomes expected with the practice change.

A pilot project among a small number of units that is limited in size and scope allows practice change leaders to carefully assess strategies employed in the practice change, get feedback, and improve the change process as needed to enhance outcome effectiveness or adherence to processes (Green & Seifert, 2005). When unit personnel are amenable to change with alterations in the original plan, and are asked for feedback and decisions about changes needed, they become clinical champions and can be educators and informal leaders when widespread implementation occurs. If choosing a pilot unit over widespread implementation, before moving to widespread implementation, leaders should consider if patient populations, nursing personnel number and type, or other factors will alter the implementation and quality monitoring plan. When the population studied in research is different from the population in which the practice change is being implemented, it is important to carefully assess clinical and administrative outcomes to ensure project goals are realized. Finally, small pilot projects can be costly and can cause disruption in services between units, especially when nurses float to other units or services and equipment are expected to be shared. Leaders need to anticipate issues that could emerge due to practice-environment factors and also among laggard adopters who may not embrace the practice change.

Translate by Conducting Research

An alternative to translating research by implementing a practice change is to translate research by implementing a real-world pragmatic research study of the research intervention, so that generalizability of research findings can be determined and fine-tuned. It is common to translate experimental research by conducting clinical research. For example, basic science (animal testing) research is frequently translated into phase 1 research that may involve testing in a limited number of humans to determine overall safety, then into phase 2 research that involves dosing or prescribing of the new intervention (efficacy), and then into phase 3 research that involves assessment of intervention effectiveness in a randomized, controlled trial. When nurses translate research by conducting research, the goal may be to support behavior change among clinicians. Some inclusion and exclusion criteria from the original research may be omitted (e.g., older age, minority status, renal dysfunction, end-of-life status) and the intervention may be tailored to overcome factors that could impair clinical use or effectiveness. Translation of research findings by conducting new research may be targeted to improve patient–clinician communication, care coordination, clinician training, or may have a goal of eliminating waste or promoting continuous quality assessment and improvement efforts.

Translation by conducting research is an important strategy when the original research involved determining predictors of risk or assessing a new process/device to a gold standard. A derivation study leads to important new knowledge; however, findings should be confirmed in a validation study. Further, research that had a great effect but had limitations and biases due to being single-centered; having a small, homogeneous sample; or utilizing one research coordinator who might be a factor in the success of the intervention requires further research before translation via implementation of practice change.

Monitoring and Evaluating Practice Changes Reflecting Research Translation

Whenever practice changes are implemented, it is important to monitor and evaluate the effectiveness of integration of new knowledge into existing knowledge. A shift in context requires methods that reinforce new knowledge and new practices. Simulations that involve exposure to new knowledge and practice changes can be used as a scaffold to integration, but most commonly, health care organizations use quality improvement models to monitor and evaluate practice changes or expected outcomes of practice changes as shown in Figure 8.1.

The amount of time required to attend to practice changes will be based on multiple factors. The complexity of new knowledge and procedural steps may require more deliberate practice (repetition) to attain expert performance (Green & Seifert, 2005). If time is taken up front to tailor interventions to overcome barriers to change, monitoring time may be reduced (Titler, 2007). Further, refinement of performance through quality assessment and user feedback may lengthen the amount of attentive time required to ensure translation goals are met.

CONCLUSION

Translation of new knowledge gained through research is an important aspect of research work that is time consuming and often fraught with complexity. Nurse researchers should coach nurse investigators in determining if translation into clinical practice or into another research study is the best translation approach. Nurse researchers should consider the multiple factors discussed about characteristics of new knowledge, communication processes, social systems, users of the new knowledge, stakeholders, and cost analysis when determining an implementation plan. Finally, monitoring and evaluation for optimal and effective adoption of practice changes will strengthen use of high quality evidence-based nursing practices.

REFERENCES

Agency for Healthcare Research and Quality. (2001). *Translating Research Into Practice (TRIP)-II*. AHRQ Pub No. 01-P017. Retrieved from http://archive.ahrq.gov/research/findings/factsheets/translating/tripfac/trip2fac.pdf

Benner, P. (1984). *From novice to expert: Excellence and power in clinical nursing practice.* Menlo Park, CA: Addison Wesley.

Bradley, E. H., Webster, T. R., Baker, D., Schlesinger, M., Inouye, S. K., Barth, M., . . . Koren, M. J. (2004). Translating research into practice: Speeding the adoption of innovative heath care programs. *Issue Brief (The Commonwealth Fund), 724*, 1–12.

Clark, A. M., & Thompson, D. R. (2014). "I don't have enough time . . .": Myths and strategies for implementing academic workplace effectiveness. *Nursing Outlook, 62*, 231–234. doi: 10.1016/j.outlook.2014.06.002

Davis, D. A., & Taylor-Vaisey, A. (1997). Translating guidelines into practice. *Canadian Medical Association Journal, 157*, 408–416.

Dearmon, V., Roussel, L., Buckner, E. B., Mulekar, M., Pomrenke, B., Salas, S., . . . Brown, A. (2013). Transforming care at the bedside (TCAB): Enhancing direct care and value-added care. *Journal of Nursing Management, 21*, 668–678. doi: 10.1111/j.1365-2834.2012.01412.x

Farquhar, C. M., Stryer, D., & Slutsky, J. (2002). Translating research into practice: The future ahead. *International Journal for Quality in Health Care, 14*, 233–249.

Green, L. A., & Seifert, C. M. (2005). Translation of research into practice: Why we can't "just do it." *Journal of the American Board of Family Medicine, 18*, 541–545.

Grimshaw, J. M., Eccles, M. P., Lavis, J. N., Hill, S. J., & Squires, J. E. (2012). Knowledge translation of research findings. *Implementation Science, 7*, 50. doi: 10.1186/1748-5908-7-50

Gruen, R. L., Elliott, J. H., Nolan, M. L., Lawton, P. D., Parkhill, A., McLaren, C. J., & Lavis, J. N. (2008). Sustainability science: An integrated approach for health-programme planning. *Lancet, 372*, 1579–1589. doi: 10.1016/S0140-6736(08)61659-1

Khoury, M. J., Gwinn, M., & Ioannidis, J. P. (2010). The emergence of translational epidemiology: From scientific discovery to population health impact. *American Journal of Epidemiology, 172*, 517–24. doi: 10.1093/aje/kwq211

Melnyk, B. M., & Morrison-Beedy, D. (2012). *Intervention research: Designing, conducting, analyzing and funding.* New York, NY: Springer.

Morris, Z. S., Wooding, S., & Grant, J. (2011). The answer is 17 years, what is the question: Understanding time lags in translational research. *Journal of Royal Society of Medicine, 104,* 510–520. doi: 10.1258/jrsm.2011.110180

Murthy, L., Shepperd, S., Clarke, M. J., Garner, S. E., Lavis, J. N., Perrier, L., . . . Straus, S. E. (2012). Interventions to improve the use of systematic reviews in decision-making by health system managers, policy makers and clinicians. *Cochrane Database Systematic Reviews, 9*:CD009401. doi: 10.1002/14651858.CD009401.pub2

Nieva, V. F., Murphy, R., Ridley, N., Donaldson, N., Combes, J., Mitchell, P., . . . Carpenter, D. (2005). From science to service: A framework for the transfer of patient safety research into practice. In K. Henriksen, J. B. Battles, E. S. Marks, (Eds.), *Advances in patient safety: From research to implementation (Volume 2: Concepts and methodology).* Rockville, MD: Agency for Healthcare Research and Quality.

The Office of Nursing Research and Innovation, Cleveland Clinic. (2015). *Cleveland Clinic Nursing Institute translation of new knowledge into practice.* Cleveland, OH: Cleveland Clinic Foundation.

Rogers, E. (2003). *Diffusion of innovations.* (5th ed.). New York, NY: The Free Press.

Rubenstein, L. V., & Pugh, J. (2006). Strategies for promoting organizational and practice change by advancing implementation research. *Journal of General Internal Medicine, 21*(Suppl 2), S58–S64. doi: 10.1111/j.1525–1497.2006.00364.x

Titler, M. (2007). Translating research into practice. *American Journal of Nursing, 107,* 26–33. doi: 10.1097/01.NAJ.0000277823.51806.10

Ubbink, D. T., Guyatt, G. H., & Vermeulen, H. (2013). Framework of policy recommendations for implementation of evidence-based practice: A systematic scoping review. *BMJ Open, 3*(1). pii: e001881. doi: 10.1136/bmjopen-2012-001881

Unruh, L., Agrawal, M., & Hassmiller, S. (2011). The business case for transforming care at the bedside among the "TCAB 10" and lessons learned. *Nursing Administration Quarterly, 35,* 97–109. doi: 10.1097/NAQ.0b013e31820f696f

What is health care quality and who decides? Hearing before the Subcommittee on Health Care, Committee on Finance, Senate, 111th Cong. (2009) (Testimony of Carolyn M. Clancy). Retrieved from http://www.hhs.gov/asl/testify/2009/03/t20090318b.html

Jeanne Sorrell
Tonya Rutherford-Hemming

9

DISSEMINATING RESEARCH

Previous chapters emphasized the importance of implementing research to provide the best evidence for nursing practice and, thus, improve patient care. Sometimes this is referred to as knowledge transfer, or a process that promotes transfer of evidence into practice. Unless research results are transferred into practice, knowledge that comes from research is not available to guide clinical practice. Thus, the aim of knowledge transfer is to close the research-to-practice gap.

This chapter addresses the need for dissemination of research and focuses on dissemination both inside the hospital organization and outside. Disseminating results of research is often the most exciting phase of the process, as it is the culmination and highlight of countless hours of work. Sharing the results of a project for a local, regional, national, or international audience is not only "payoff" for you, the investigator, but sets the stage for others to embark on new endeavors in research based on the current state of the science. Common areas for dissemination internally include presentations to colleagues on your unit, as well as across the hospital organization. Internal presentations offer a direct way for you to provide new evidence for practice in your hospital organization. In addition, however, it is important that results of your research reach nurses and other health professionals nationally and internationally. Thus, you will want to participate in media dissemination of your research, systematically look for calls for abstracts to present at professional conferences, and disseminate your research through professional publications.

DISSEMINATING RESEARCH THROUGH PRESENTATIONS

Researchers often emphasize the importance of publication of results in peer-reviewed publications, but it is also important to realize the importance of disseminating research internally. Think about how to reach audiences that should know about your research. Many nurses may not read a research journal but would read a newsletter or attend a local research conference. Thus, it is important to consider multiple ways for effective dissemination of research to nurses. Locally, informing nurses about research results can promote positive attitudes, new knowledge, and behaviors that reflect an integration of research into clinical practice.

Newsletters

Many hospital leadership and nursing unit teams create and distribute newsletters. These may take the form of electronic informal monthly updates on changes in the hospital's organization or more formal printed documents. An example of a regularly published newsletter to engage nurses in applying research to their practice is the University of New Mexico Hospitals publication of *Research Round-up Newsletter* at hospitals.unm.edu/nursing-research/ newsletter.shtml. Another example is *Notable Nursing*, published by the Zielony Nursing Institute at the Cleveland Clinic. *Notable Nursing* features two completed research projects and two best practices in each issue, led by clinical nurses in the hospital organization (my.clevelandclinic.org/services/ nursing-institute/news-publications/publications). Another format for an online newsletter is the *Sacred Cow Campaign* initiated by the Cleveland Clinic's main campus Nursing Research Council to encourage nurses to think about "sacred cow" rituals that were implemented without evidence of effectiveness. Online communications engage nurses to discuss use of interventions that may need to be "put out to pasture" (Figure 9.1).

Journal Clubs

Many hospitals have journal clubs where nurses meet regularly to review research papers. This is an excellent way to help generate both knowledge and interest in research. Reading a published research study and then discussing its application in practice, as well as critiquing the research methodology used, can stimulate nurses to consider how they can use the evidence in their practice, and whether they need additional evidence to determine best practices. Journal clubs are also a good time to discuss plans for new research projects and generate ideas about how to design and implement them effectively.

Unit Meetings and Postings

Informal meetings and posted notices on nursing units can be effective ways to help nurses learn about new research results that have a potential impact on clinical practice. Clinical nurses may have difficultly breaking away from

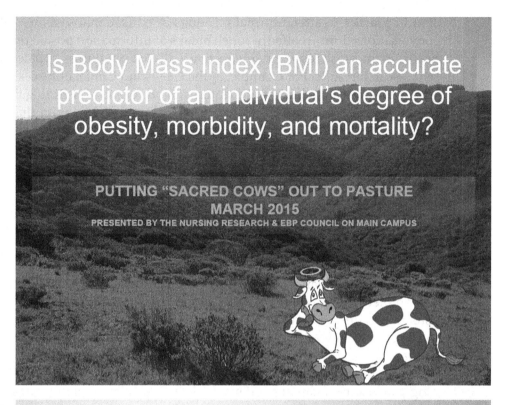

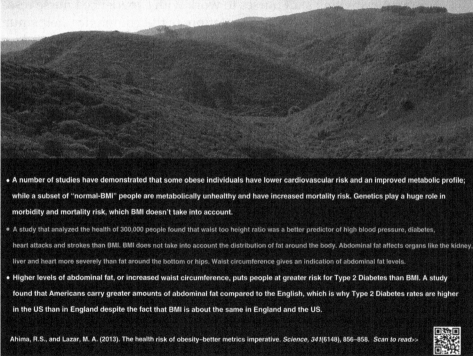

FIGURE 9.1 Putting "sacred cows" out to pasture.

clinical practice to attend formal meetings or educational sessions. Informal conversations during coffee or lunch breaks or information posted on bulletin boards in the break room can be effective ways to keep nurses updated on current research results. For example, at the Cleveland Clinic, unit-based nurses who are diabetes management mentors attend formal classes to gain knowledge about recent research related to the care of patients with diabetes. In turn, they are responsible for sharing this information with nurses on their unit. They plan fun, easy-to-access activities, such as games or self-assessment quizzes, to communicate information about new evidence that can be used to improve care for patients with diabetes.

Institution-Wide Conferences

Many hospitals, small and large, hold annual nursing conferences that focus on completed research or evidence-based practice (EBP) projects. Research conferences offer wonderful opportunities for showcasing completed nursing research that was translated into practice at the hospital organization, as well as informing attendees of new evidence that may impact their practice. Research conference dissemination requires extensive planning, and the planning process itself can engage nurses in learning more about research. For example, inviting staff nurses to work with experienced nurse researchers to select abstracts for oral presentation at the conference helps nurses learn about what should be included in an abstract and the strength and weaknesses of different types of evidence.

External Research Presentations

As nurses become more knowledgeable about research and EBP and implement their own projects, it is important to consider disseminating evidence outside the hospital organization. Research presentations through the media and at professional conferences are an important part of professional practice. The following information presented can help you prepare for these activities.

Dissemination of Research Through Media

Newspaper, radio, and television journalists are often good resources to help disseminate research results. Contact the marketing department at your hospital organization to let them know about currently active or completed nursing research that would be of interest to the public. This is an excellent way to market innovative work at your hospital organization and is a valuable professional experience in communicating with the lay public. Your marketing contact may request an interview to learn more about your research. Think about how to concisely communicate the most important aspects of your research to the public. Did you use a new methodology? Were your results surprising? How do your results relate to previous research on the same topic? Often there is very limited time during an interview but you can prepare an "elevator speech" to communicate important sound-bites in only a few minutes.

Dissemination of Research via Conference Presentation
Many research conferences send out a "call for abstracts" several months to a year before the planned conference. Preplanning provides nurses with a time line that allows for data collection and analysis before the deadline. Abstract deadlines also assist the sponsoring hospital organization, as a review team will determine the best studies to select for the conference. Usually, only completed studies are eligible for abstract submission and presentation. Wait until your data are analyzed and implications are known before sending an abstract for consideration at a conference.

You may find calls for abstracts in journals that are associated with professional organizations. Most journals are accessible online through library databases. Many professional organizations send the request to submit abstracts directly to members. Nursing organizations such as the American Nurses Association (ANA) and Sigma Theta Tau International (STTI) have conferences throughout each year, providing excellent opportunities for reaching broad and diverse audiences. Geographically based nursing research organizations such as the Midwest Nursing Research Society (MNRS) and Southern Nursing Research Society (SNRS) have annual conferences that include poster and podium presentations. In addition, local hospital organizations in close proximity to your workplace may invite research abstracts.

Once a conference venue is selected for your research presentation, consider the feasibility of traveling. Are travel expenses reimbursable? Is the registration fee reimbursable? If the hospital organization cannot pay for all expenses, can you negotiate expenses reimbursement or will you cover the charges yourself? Many hospitals fund travel for professional presentations within the country but not international travel. There may be a cap on airfare or hotel room rates that you should consider in advance. Feasibility also includes checking the hospital or nursing department calendar to be sure you are able to be away from your hospital organization on the conference dates. It is considered unprofessional to submit an abstract, allow it to be accepted, and then cancel attendance and presentation. Consider that other abstracts may have been rejected so yours could be accepted. If you develop a pattern of submitting abstracts and then canceling attendance due to financial constraints or because you were hoping to present your paper orally and only were accepted as a poster presenter, organization meeting planners may stop accepting your work. Of course, unpredictable events that cause a cancellation of conference attendance plans are unavoidable but consider home and work factors before submitting.

Writing a Research Abstract

A research abstract is a short, comprehensive summary of the main elements of your research study. A well-written abstract can make a difference in receiving acceptance to present results at a professional conference. Reviewers will form an initial opinion of the strength of your research based on your written words so it is very important to be as clear and as descriptive as possible within the word or character limitations.

Carefully read the instructions for writing an abstract. Your abstract has the best chance of acceptance if you follow the guidelines provided in the call for abstracts notice. If abstract guidelines specify a maximum of 300 words, you must stay within that word limit; otherwise your abstract may not be considered. Conferences usually receive many more abstracts than they can accept and may automatically eliminate those that do not meet specified guidelines. Figure 9.2 shows a typical call for abstracts.

Since abstracts are short documents, many people assume they are easy to write, but that is a fallacy. Include enough detail so that readers gain a clear understanding of the value of the research results. Due to space limitations, specific topics of discussion, especially secondary aims, may need to be excluded. Abstract rewriting before submission is common, as is sharing with others for feedback. Therefore, leave enough time before the submission deadline for rewriting.

Most abstract guidelines have headings, as suggested in Figure 9.2. If abstract guidelines do not have specific headings or sections, you can add heading words to make your abstract clearer; for example, start the conclusion with: "In conclusion. . . ." Questions that an abstract should answer are: What was done? What was found? What does it mean (implications)? Due to limited space, write only one or two sentences for each section of the abstract, except "results," where more content is generally needed. For example, create one sentence for the background and one sentence for the purpose. Often, writers spend too much time on the background or context and not enough on the methods or results sections of the abstract. Make every word count, and be specific. Under the results and implications subheadings, do not say "results will be discussed" or "implications of research will be presented"; provide specific results and implications that relate to the research. Reviewers need to understand the fit between the purpose of the research, methods, results, and implications. Figures 9.3 and 9.4 present abstracts of qualitative and quantitative research that were accepted for a research conference, and Table 9.1 provides general points to consider when developing an abstract.

Once a final draft of your abstract is completed and you are certain that it is within the maximum word limit and has all the required subsections, have more than one colleague review the draft to make suggestions for changes. Your engagement in the research process creates familiarity of study details, but written words may be unclear to readers who have not been as closely involved. Thus, it is helpful to seek reviewers who are not familiar with the

Provide all information requested below and send electronically to Dr. Jane Doe, Research Coordinator, at JDoe@ehospital.edu. Abstracts must be received by month-day-year to be considered for acceptance. You will receive a confirmation once your abstract is received. You should receive a notice of abstract acceptance by month-day-year.

Submissions must describe clinically relevant research, empirical evaluations of clinical innovations, or development of research instruments for clinical research. Submissions will be selected based upon their relevance and appropriateness for the target audience of nurses engaged in clinical practice.

Information for Abstract Submission

The body of all abstracts should have a maximum of xxx words (or xxxx characters, including spaces)

1. Names, titles, and organizational affiliation of all investigators

2. Name, address, telephone, and e-mail for a contact person

3. Title of research study

4. Abstract of project to include: not all abstract submittal systems require the same headers, but all will include the four primary headers: Background, Methods, Results, Conclusions/Implications.

    (a) Purpose

    (b) Background/significance

    (c) Theoretical or Conceptual Framework: not all abstract submittal systems require the same headers, but all will include the four primary headers: Background, Methods, Results, Conclusions/Implications.

    (d) Sample

    (e) Methods

    (f) Results

    (g) Conclusions/Implications

FIGURE 9.2 Call for abstracts.

study, as they can make suggestions that increase clarity, succinctness, and completeness. Have your statistician review the research analysis methods and results sections. Suggested edits may increase the accuracy of the analysis plan and results. Also, make sure that there are no spelling or grammar errors. When abstracts have errors, reviewers may think the researchers are careless or may wonder if they can trust the research results.

There are some ethical concerns to consider when submitting abstracts. Most conference organizers assume that an abstract has been submitted solely to them, and that the abstract is not one part of a research study with multiple components or outcomes that should really be presented in one abstract, rather than parsed into many abstracts, and sent to many conferences. Please review abstract guidelines carefully. If abstract guidelines state that they accept previously presented research, then it is okay to resubmit

Qualitative Research

Creating Expertise With a Diabetes Management Mentor Program:

Doing the Right Thing for the Right Reason

Purpose: This qualitative research study explored the research question: What is the lived experience of Diabetic Management Mentors in implementing the mentoring role?

Background/Significance: A Diabetes Management Mentor program was implemented to meet the critical need for enhancing competence of nurses in caring for hospitalized patients with diabetes.

Theoretical Framework: Anthony Weston's framework was used, in which ethical practice is guided by broad categories of practical intelligence required in moral judgment, which expands the traditional principle-based approaches to ethics.

Sample: Participants included 12 Diabetes Management Mentors on 10 different units of a large academic health care center in the Midwest.

Methods: A phenomenological approach was used for data collection and analysis. After IRB approval, interviews with Diabetes Management Mentors were audiotaped and transcribed verbatim. Data were analyzed with van Manen's approach through collaborative coding of interviews to identify themes.

Results: One striking theme was *Doing the Right Thing for the Right Reason*, which illustrated the practical intelligence that is needed for moral judgment in making ethical decisions related to practice. Other salient themes included *Making a Difference in Safety for Acutely Ill Patients With Diabetes* and *Using Knowledge to Change the Culture of Practice*. Stories from participants revealed that Diabetes Management Mentors frequently stepped in to guide peers in ethical practice by standing firm when confronted with orders or practices that would have resulted in suboptimal care and even dangerous errors.

Conclusions/Implications: It was evident from participants' stories that the unique curriculum and ongoing development of the Diabetes Management Mentor program enhance mentors' knowledge, confidence, and tenacity to model exemplary professional practice and help to ensure ethical comportment in caring for hospitalized patients with diabetes.

FIGURE 9.3 An example of an accepted abstract.

previously presented work, but that still does not mean that a newly created abstract can be submitted to more than one conference at a time. Of note, presentations delivered at the hospital organization responsible for the research are considered internal presentations and are not subject to the duplicate submission rule. Make sure that all authors who are listed with your abstract submission participated in the research. Some conferences require that anyone listed as an author attend the conference or disclose their role in the research project, so it is important to determine authorship before submission. Further, ensure that all listed authors meet the criteria for authorship; generally, they must have intellectual property in the research by assisting with the study design, data collection, analysis, or implications. Be prepared to identify any potential or actual conflicts of interest regarding research implementation; for example, research that was externally funded by an organization, government, or corporation grant, even if the specific research theme does not contain content that could be considered biased.

Quantitative Research

Nurse Practitioner Students' Perceived Self-Efficacy With Standardized Patient Simulation

Background/Purpose: The purpose of this proposed study was to investigate the issue of transfer of learning of knowledge and skills by observing students in a standardized patient simulation and then in clinical practice. This study sought to learn if nurse practitioner students who participated in a simulation experience with standardized patients prior to entering their first clinical rotation demonstrated an increase in clinical competency in the clinical practice setting. It also sought to learn if students who participated in a simulation experience with standardized patients prior to entering their clinical practicum showed increases in perceived self-efficacy.

Methods: The present study used a descriptive research design with 14 nurse practitioner students who participated in a standardized patient simulation. Students were observed in the simulation setting and in the clinical setting, and they evaluated their own perceived self-efficacy at three points during the study (prior to the simulation, after the simulation, and prior to seeing the first patient in the clinical setting).

Results: Results from the study indicated that overall there was increased growth in students' competency scores from Time 1 (in the simulation laboratory) to Time 2 (in the clinical setting; $p < .05$). In addition, there was an overall statistically significant correlation between the competency scores of students in the simulation lab (Time 1) and the competency scores of the same students in the clinical setting (Time 2; $p < .05$). While students' overall self-efficacy scores increased over time, the mean scores did not change significantly across time.

Conclusions: While there is a sense that simulation improves learning opportunities, little is known about the processes that students use to integrate such learning into their ongoing practice. Little is also known about the direct clinical translation of simulated skills into clinical settings in nurse practitioner education. This study represents one of the first systematic investigations of the processes by which students transfer simulated skills into direct clinical practice.

Relevance to Conference Themes: It contributes to the understanding of effective instructional methods and provides guidance to faculty using simulation technology, supporting both process and program improvement.

FIGURE 9.4 An example of an accepted abstract.

Choosing Poster Versus Podium Presentation

During the submittal process for your abstract, there may be an option regarding presentation preference: poster or podium (oral) presentation. Deciding between poster and podium presentation can be difficult. Novice presenters may feel uneasy, unprepared, and anxious about presenting in front of a large crowd or feel unprepared to answer questions from the audience. Poster presentations allow for one-on-one and small group discussions. Many nurses find that presenting research in a poster format is an enjoyable way to become familiar with presenting research results at professional conferences, helps conquer a fear of public speaking, and builds confidence that will help later when leading podium presentations.

Research Poster Presentations

Poster sessions are commonly organized at conferences to accommodate a large number of abstracts of new research knowledge that would not be able to be included due to limited podium time available. Since many conferences set up poster presentations to be viewed and discussed only during

TABLE 9.1 Points to Consider When Writing an Abstract

General	• Follow the posted guidelines for word/character count and use of tables or figures. • No abbreviations without writing out the first time. • No abbreviations in the title. • Be careful of use of "symbols"; some submittal systems will alter them. • All parts of the abstract must match. Do not introduce new themes in the results or implications (conclusion) sections that were not introduced in the background or methods sections. • Do not provide proper names of data collection sites; use geographical area and hospital characteristics; see Figure 9.3. • No quotes. • No references.
Title	• Keep it short; generally 10 to 12 words or less. • If a multicenter study, say so. • If a randomized controlled study, say so. • Okay to be clever with wording, but use medical subject heading terms whenever possible and be sure the reader can tell what the abstract is about from the title alone.
Background	• Be simple and concise—generally one sentence in length. • Tell the reader why he or she should care about this topic.
Purpose or Objective	• Be concise—generally one sentence in length. • Do not include content that belongs in the methods section, such as setting or sample, research design, tools used, or analysis methods.
Methods	• The first sentence should convey the study design and may also include the setting, sample, intervention, when applicable, and study outcomes. One sentence should provide analysis methods. • If space is available, may include measurement methods of independent and dependent variables.
Results	• The first sentence should convey the sample size and brief demographics so the reader can determine if the sample matches the target population in characteristics. • Provide results of primary study purpose/aim/hypothesis. • If space is available, provide results of secondary analysis. • If multivariable or multivariate analyses were performed, provide results before providing univariate results. Only provide both if space allows. • Retain ordering of independent and dependent variables in the results section, to match what was written in the table, purpose and methods sections. • Show p values if space allows.
Conclusion	• Be concise and provide the main study results without statistics in the first sentence. • Be careful not to overstate results. • If space is available, provide one sentence on implications to clinical nursing practice; again, do not overstate implications.

designated time periods, attendees often move quickly from poster to poster. When presenting research by a poster, consider the most important talking points reflecting research results and implications. Refine and polish an "elevator speech" in preparation for discussion with conference attendees.

Once an abstract is accepted for a poster presentation at a conference, review presentation guidelines related to poster size and whether it will be freestanding on a table or easel or whether it will be pinned on a display board. Most conferences want posters to be a standard size, such as 3×6 feet. If your hospital organization does not have poster creation and printing services, a commercial printer can be used at most office supply or printing stores at a cost of several hundred dollars. Freestanding poster content is contained on a flat or tri-fold poster board, or content may be printed on heavy, flexible paper and pinned to a display board. Tubes to transport flexible posters are available at office supply stores; they are inexpensive and help protect posters during travel. Fabric (silk) printing is also available but is more expensive than paper printing. Benefits of a fabric poster are that it may be more durable for presenting research results at multiple conferences. Also, it is convenient to fold a fabric poster and place it in luggage, rather than carry it in a separate tube. Generally, fabric posters do not wrinkle.

Preparing your poster is both a scholarly and a creative process. Some hospital organizations may have an art department with personnel who use special software to prepare a poster once the content has been developed, but it is not uncommon for research nurses to prepare the poster content in totality themselves. Learn if the hospital organization has a poster template that may include the hospital logo and may require a specific style or coloring. A preformatted template will save time and help ensure professional representation of your work. Plan poster content carefully to include all pertinent information about the research study and to have aesthetic appeal. What colors are best to use? How large should the font be? What types of pictures or graphs should be used? Table 9.2 provides poster creation points adapted from DeSilets (2010).

Poster content is divided into sections that are similar to the abstract: purpose, background/significance, theoretical/conceptual framework (when requested), methods (generally includes setting, sample, independent and dependent variables, measurement, data collection and analysis), results, and conclusions/implications. Microsoft PowerPoint software may be used to prepare poster content, especially if hospital organization services are not available to prepare and print a poster. It is helpful to use the ruler or gridlines function in PowerPoint to ensure that different sections of the poster are aligned evenly. Before taking a poster to the printer, authors should review content for accuracy, completeness, and aesthetics. When using a hospital organization resource to prepare and print posters, generally the content is prepared in a Word document. A template can be created to ensure optimal spacing, white spaces, and text length based on the poster size. Figure 9.5

TABLE 9.2 Points to Consider in Developing a Research Poster

General	• What do you want the take-home message to be for your audience?
	• Make your poster information clear, readable, and visually attractive to capture and maintain viewers' attention.
	• Use fonts that are easily read (e.g., a sans serif font).
	• Be conservative with the variety of fonts you use. Just because you can use a variety doesn't mean you should.
	• Keep labels and captions brief.
	• Use boldface, underlining, italics, all capital letters, and Word Art selectively to make words or headings stand out and identify key information.
	• Generally, use at least a 36-point font for text and a 48-point font for the title.
	• Viewers should be able to read your poster from a distance of 4 to 8 feet.
	• Information should flow from left to right, top to bottom.
	• 3×6 foot posters generally have three columns; 3×8 foot posters generally have four columns; and 4×4 foot posters generally have two columns below the title, authors, and hospital organization area.
	• Simplify wording; be concise, precise, and straightforward.
	• Avoid jargon; identify the meaning of all acronyms and use sparingly.
	• Condense ideas and focus on central themes. Show what you did, why you did it, and what it contributes to a body of knowledge.
	• Use colors appropriately. Contrasting colors work well. Warm colors are thought to be inviting.
	• Use at least a 150 to 300 dpi resolution for pictures. Include a caption for each graphic.
	• Consider branding your poster with a logo or colors from your hospital organization.
	• Do not put too much information on your poster. Leave some white space.
	• Communicate your main points quickly and clearly. Ask yourself if each item on the poster adds to what you are trying to communicate.
Title and Authors	• Keep the title brief; use key words.
	• The title should provide enough detail about the study to draw attention to your poster.
	• Include the names, city, and state of each author.
Abstract	• If the poster is busy, OK to use smaller font or delete the abstract
Background	• Two to five bullets that introduce the research theme and include a conceptual or theoretical model, if used.
	• One bullet on the study purpose; place research questions immediately before the methods section.
Methods	• Use subheaders to convey the design, setting and sample, intervention, outcomes and measurement, data collection methods, and data analysis.
	• In the design subheader, include one bullet on institutional review board (IRB) approval.
Results	• Use figures and tables to convey results. Many statistical analysis programs produce figures and graphs that can be embedded.
	■ Clearly label x and y axes and create a legend if needed for abbreviations and descriptors.
	■ In tables, always include the unit of measure for each data point.
	• Do not replicate content from figures and tables in text.
Limitations	• Every research study has limitations—use bullets to convey.
Conclusion and References	• Do not overstate conclusions. Stay focused on your research.
	• If the poster is busy, okay to use a smaller font in the references
	• Acknowledgments should be placed at the end of the poster (lower right corner) and should include funding sources.

IRB, institutional review board.

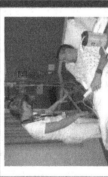

FIGURE 9.5 Poster (6') example with good density.

197

presents a poster with good use of text and black space. Figure 9.6 presents a poster with more information; its denseness might make it more difficult to read unless standing very close. This poster has a lot of information but would not have as high an appeal to conference participants with limited time to review posters.

Before arriving at the conference, review the date(s) when the poster should be displayed, the poster number assigned, and hours assigned to put up and take down posters. This information is usually available in your acceptance letter and conference syllabus. Many conference organizers include specific hours for poster presentation with the primary presenter at each poster, ready to discuss it with conference attendees, even if they want posters displayed throughout the conference. If a display board is used, pushpins are usually provided, but read the acceptance letter carefully. Dress professionally, with comfortable shoes, as there may be periods of extended standing. Bring business cards so that viewers can contact you for further information. Consider providing a supplemental handout; for example, 8.5×14 inch or 11×17 inch paper versions of the poster, or a reference list to enhance the research presentation.

Engage viewers in conversation about the research as they pass by your poster. Poster presentations are often passive; knowledge transfer will be enhanced by dialogue with viewers about key aspects of the research (Ilic & Rowe, 2013). Prior to the conference date, practice summarizing the research results in one or two sentences, to convey the essence of the research without overwhelming viewers with details (McClendon & Stover, 2014). Poster presenters should look attentive and welcoming of questions without hovering over poster viewers. Standing to one side of the poster avoids blocking information, yet it allows for eye contact with poster viewers, which may encourage questions and exchange of ideas. Others who walk by and observe animated interactions may be drawn into discussion (McClendon & Stover, 2014). Conversing with poster viewers has many rewards. It may lead to constructive feedback regarding strengths and limitations of the research design or results. Viewers may offer suggestions for translation into clinical practice or provide evidence of similar research results that expand the generalizability of the current research. Viewers may make suggestions for ways to expand the research theme, offer suggestions for subanalyses, or offer information about their own research that helps in research interpretation and implications.

Poster presentations take a lot of planning and also bring many benefits. Poster presentations can enhance speaking skills and increase recognition of common questions about the research topic that will be useful when presenting in larger venues in the future. A completed research poster may be used for evidence of professional development, as part of a clinical ladder portfolio (Durkin, 2011). Perhaps most important, the experience of presenting a poster at a professional conference can help poster authors realize the value of their research and its potential to improve nursing practice and patient care.

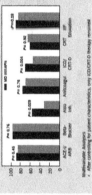

FIGURE 9.6 Poster (6') with higher content density.

VOICES OF NURSE RESEARCHERS

Karen Johnson, PhD, RN
Director, Nursing Research, Banner Health, Phoenix, Arizona

We developed dissemination/presentation guidelines to help staff through the poster presentation process. We require manager approval (for proprietary review) and then review by a director of professional practice or clinical nurse specialist (for quality review). This really serves as an internal peer review process and as a record-keeping process so that we can track external dissemination. We also developed poster templates for process improvement, evidence-based practice (EBP), and research so that our posters would look uniform and professional. The poster template serves as a tutorial as well.

Laura McNicholl, RN-BC, MS, CNS-BC
Vicki Lindgren, RN, MSN, CNS, CCRN, CCNS
Clinical Nurse Specialists, Inova Fair Oaks Hospital, Fairfax, Virginia

In 2011, it was noted that our utilization rates for urinary catheters were above the National Healthcare Safety Network (NHSN) benchmarks, placing our patients at a risk for developing catheter-associated urinary tract infections. We developed and implemented an evidence-based practice (EBP) nurse-driven protocol to remove urinary catheters and completed a pilot on two units. In 2014, we had encouragement from the system nursing research and EBP coordinator to submit a poster to a state conference. We submitted an abstract and got accepted! The coordinator shared the health system posters template with us. The poster was easier than expected with the template. This same poster was displayed at two other nursing conferences that year and then updated and shared at another state conference in 2015. Sometimes you just need a little nudge of encouragement from a colleague to get you moving in the right direction.

Research Podium Presentations
Oral presentations at a podium are an excellent venue for broad dissemination of research. Since oral presentations are generally limited by space on the conference schedule, abstracts that ranked highest when peer-reviewed are more likely to be selected. Thus, oral presentations are often viewed as more prestigious than poster presentations, and employers may expect or require podium

presentations for promotion of image or branding. Podium presentations may be delivered in a large general conference session or within smaller breakout sessions. Regardless of the audience size, podium presentations provide a captive audience. Delivery of content should be carefully planned. Effective delivery of research methods, results, and implications will keep an audience interested and entertained, and interested and entertained audiences are more likely to remember the information being delivered.

Understand the audience before developing a podium presentation (Greenhalgh, de Jongste, & Brand, 2011; Longo & Tierney, 2012). If the audience is composed of mostly novices, dedicate additional time in the beginning of the presentation to more detailed background information so the audience fully appreciates the rationale for the study and the results. Further, an audience of primarily novice research nurses may not understand how to interpret slides with statistical analyses details or figures and tables that depict research results. When the slides are presented, it might be important to orient the audience to important visual details. If the audience members are experienced researchers, allotting extra time for discussion at the end of the presentation may make the presentation memorable. In either situation, you are more likely to lose the audience's interest when you are not familiar with their expectations and if the presentation is not polished.

PowerPoint is a staple of most podium presentations. Guidelines about how to develop a professional PowerPoint presentation are available (Greenhalgh, de Jongste, & Brand, 2011; Hoffman & Mittleman, 2004; Longo & Tierney, 2012; Yang, 2010). Table 9.3 provides points in developing a PowerPoint research presentation. PowerPoint slides provide visual information to supplement oral narration but too much written text on a slide makes it difficult for the audience to determine which points are more important. Be selective and do not write in full sentences; use bullets. If you "read" your presentation directly from slides, word for word, the audience will lose interest.

PowerPoint does not have to be used in podium presentations unless required by the sponsoring conference organization. This format may leave the audience to passively absorb the presentation. As the expert, decide the best tools to use to present content. Presentation tools other than PowerPoint include flipcharts, DVDs, and various types of props (Longo & Tierney, 2012). Simple or creative handouts can also be advantageous in helping to engage the audience.

If you need presentation notes, type or write notes that are large enough to be read in a darkened room and without squinting or having to make awkward pauses. In some conference centers, there may not be a podium in each meeting room to place notes, thus, do not plan to read notes to the audience; only refer to the notes occasionally. Reading notes reflects being unprepared and not the expert of your topic (which you are!).

When developing a podium presentation, have a strong opening to attract the audience's attention (DeVan & Baum, 2013). Begin your presentation by telling the audience what you want to accomplish; often these are the research

TABLE 9.3 Tips for Developing a PowerPoint Research Presentation

Background	• Determine the type of background that is appropriate for your audience. • Consider a plain background with the logo of your hospital organization. • Learn if your hospital organization has a background template ▪ A dark background with light, bright colored text or a light background with dark text are both effective.

Slides	• Include the research presentation title and all research authors and credentials.
	• The second slide is generally reserved for disclosures. Provide all potential and actual disclosures related to the research topic.
	• Funding may be placed on the second slide (as a disclosure) or the last slide (as an acknowledgment).
	• If there are only a few authors and no funding, you may place author job titles and/or employers on slide one, next to the names.
	• Titles of next slides should follow the headers of the abstract:
	  ▪ Background or introduction.
	  ▪ Purpose, aim, research questions or hypothesis.
	  ▪ Research methods (setting, sample, intervention when applicable, outcomes and measurement, independent variables and measurement, data analysis plan).
	  ▪ Results.
	  ▪ Study limitations and study conclusions.
	• Within each header, be concise. Bullets are "points," not chapters. Too many words on a slide will make it difficult for audiences to follow your ideas.
	• Keep font size and style standard for each slide.
	  ▪ Titles should be 36 to 44 point font size.
	  ▪ A font size of 32 to 34 point works well for subcategories.
	  ▪ Explanatory text should use font size 28 to 32 point.
	  ▪ Any font size less than 24 point is too small to be easily read from a distance.
	  ▪ A san serif or Arial font works well for all text.
	• Don't overuse animations (words flying in, fading, or disappearing).
	• Include references and research acknowledgments on the last slide.

Images	• Use high quality images and graphs. • Many statistical analysis programs produce figures and graphs that can be embedded in slides.
Timing	• Review and thematic presentations devote approximately 1 minute to each slide, are 10 minutes in length, and generally have less discussion per slide; therefore, devote approximately 1 minute per slide if they are mostly text and 30 seconds per slide if there are a lot of results slides that do not require discussion, just simple presentation. • Practice narrating each slide so that the presentation length is on target. • It is essential to stay within your time limit! • If too long, decrease content in the background section so that presentation of results can receive adequate time.

goals or objectives (DeVan & Baum, 2013; Longo & Tierney, 2012). Then, plan to present the main points of your research. Be selective in how much content is presented so that the time allotment is followed. Conclude the presentation by summarizing the main points of the research results or providing research implications. In this way, the audience hears the key points of the research presentation several times, and may be more likely to remember highlights.

Ending the presentation with a concrete close is as important as beginning the presentation with a strong opening. Examples of a strong conclusion are to provide a call to action (DeVan & Baum, 2013), straw poll, or notable quotation.

Novice research nurses should practice their presentations in advance by themselves and in front of a nurse researcher to increase confidence with presenting orally. Ask for honest feedback about presentation effectiveness. Nurse researchers should ask questions and prepare novice research nurses in how to field questions they cannot answer due to unavailable data, unfamiliarity with the theme of the question, or lack of knowledge about sophisticated research analyses.

Presentation rehearsal has several advantages, including helping to build confidence and improve speech and diction. Speaking skills can be learned and mastered (Yand, 2011). Rehearsing aloud allows you to find the best places in your presentation to pause, tell a story, or allow for questions. Rehearsing aloud allows you to use and hear voice inflections, and practice difficult or awkward words or phrases. Through rehearsal, you can focus on behaviors, body language (eye contact and stance), and enthusiasm (DeVan & Baum, 2013; Hoffman & Mittelman, 2004).

Rehearsal also helps to ensure delivery of research content in the allotted time period. Often when presenters are short on time, they compensate by speaking faster, and the quality of the presentation suffers. The audience may become irritated by the lack of preparation or exclusion of important points due to time constraints. Exceeding the time limit is unfair to presenters scheduled to speak later, as they may need to shorten their presentations or the discussion section may need to be limited. Anticipate a time problem if your presentation is scheduled last in a group of presenters. Often podium presentations have moderators to keep presenters on time. Moderators help ensure that all presenters are treated equally.

In case your presentation time is limited, be prepared to decrease the length of your presentation by leaving out nonessential points, especially those related to background content, but still ensure a clear presentation. When planning the presentation, allow time for questions and answers. In general, a 1-hour presentation should include 50 minutes of presentation and 10 minutes for questions and answers. Podium presentations at research conferences are often scheduled for 15 to 20 minutes, including a 5-minute question and answer period. Sometimes 2 minutes are added to exchange slides and introduce new speakers.

The date for the conference arrives and you are ready to finally present research results! You may feel nervous, but remember, you are the "expert" on the topic, and preparation and rehearsal will increase presentation effectiveness. Dress comfortably and professionally. Black, navy, gray, or other dark colors are preferable to busy prints. After arriving at the conference, find the presentation room and observe its size, podium location in relation to the screen, use of plasma monitors or computers to see the slides, pointer availability, length of the room, seating arrangement, and use of floor microphones for audience questions. Make sure an audio-visual person provides information on how to access the slides on the computer and advance them. Pay attention to how easy it is to see the screen on which slides will be projected from the podium. Note if more than one screen is used, as you will be better prepared to face both screens at various times in the presentation, rather than just focusing on one half of the room. Have a glass of water at hand in case your mouth gets dry. Make eye contact with the audience. When speakers become overly focused on delivering the presentation content, the audience is left to passively absorb it (Hoffman & Mittleman, 2004) and are more likely to become bored (Greenhalgh, de Jongste, & Brand, 2011). For a large audience in a general session of a conference, it may be harder to engage participants, but try to look at all sections of the room and make eye contact with different people in the audience. For smaller audiences, consider having some type of active hands-on learning or discussion forum as part of the presentation to help audiences move from thinking on a surface level to thinking more in-depth about the topic.

Leave time at the end of the presentation for audience questions or to make comments about the topic. If participants do not have any questions, and time is allowed, add an additional piece of information that you did not address in the presentation, or ask a question of the audience that they can respond to by a show of hands. These options allow participants to consider questions, issues, gaps in knowledge, or how the information applies in clinical practice. When participants ask questions, repeat the question. Repeating the question serves several purposes. First, it allows the entire audience to hear the question and ensures that you also heard it correctly. It provides time for you to formulate a response or consider the best response. Finally, if the session is being taped, repeating the question will enhance playback for listeners. Most audience members are silent or provide compliments on information presented; if people are critical of research methods or results, try to understand their points of view and accept them as another interpretation. Further, admitting limitations of the research or agreeing that there may be alternative explanations for research results increases others' respect for your research and for your smooth handling of controversies. Moreover, the discussion may lead to new research that advances the science of nursing. The audience attended the session because they were interested in the research topic; they want to hear your message and critique of the research process is a natural expectation, as all research has limitations. Presenters must learn not to take critiques personally.

Ultimately, podium presentations require a great deal of planning and preparation—and confidence to speak to an audience. Although it may be stressful, the question-and-answer period may provide insight into important new ideas. Also, oral presentations generally provide a larger audience than poster presentations. Research nurses may approach the presenter at the conclusion of the presentation to discuss mutual interests. Networking in this way may enhance future research on the research topic.

DISSEMINATING RESEARCH THROUGH PUBLICATION

Publication of research enhances broad dissemination with other clinicians and researchers. Writing for publication may seem like an intimidating process, but once you learn the formula for success, you are likely to find that it is not that difficult. Many times, the writing process begins by using a poster or podium presentation and revising the content and format for a manuscript for publication. There are many steps from start-up to publication, and generally, each should be carried out one at a time, so that writers do not jump ahead and get frustrated with the process.

VOICE OF A NURSE RESEARCHER

Jennifer Fabian, BSN, RN, CCRN
Staff Nurse, Intensive Care Unit, Inova Loudoun Hospital,
Leesburg, Virginia

When I became interested in participating in nursing research, I joined my hospital's Research and EBP Council. I was soon invited to be part of research studies on the topic complementary therapy of healing touch. Having no experience in conducting research, I needed much guidance in the process. As part of a team of expert researchers, nursing educators, and subject experts, I was taught how nursing research studies progress and the steps required. As a member of the research team, I was able to take part in many aspects of the nursing research process, which included obtaining consent from participants, taking notes during focus groups, assisting with theme identification in the qualitative study, and collecting data from the electronic medical record. Through the mentorship and guidance of the research team, my skills in research were developed and realized.

I have now participated in two studies on the use and implementation of healing touch in the acute care setting. As the only staff nurse on the team for one of the studies, I was in a unique position to offer suggestions about how to present the results in a clear and meaningful way for staff nurses. I feel that my most significant contribution to the team was my involvement in manuscript writing and dissemination of study findings. I provided input in writing and editing both manuscripts and assisted in creating posters for presentations within and outside of the health system. Additionally, as a means of spreading the information, I presented findings of both studies to an interprofessional team who attended the hospital's Nursing Grand Rounds presentation.

Getting Started

One of the most helpful elements to getting started with writing is to find a mentor. Nurses who have previously published research papers often enjoy helping new authors. Find someone in your hospital organization that has writing experience and a willingness to help you write a paper. You should offer potential mentors an opportunity to be a co-author, especially if they are providing intellectual property or substantive content. Not only do you gain experience in writing for publication, the mentor receives credit for supporting you toward success as a first author, as they can be listed as a senior author (the term used to depict the last author listed, who was the project mentor). Another strategy to getting started is to organize a writing support group with research colleagues and work together on different manuscripts for multiple publications.

Before writing your manuscript, determine all authors. For research papers, generally authorship includes co-investigators who invested time in the study or intellectual property. Do not forget the statistician and statistical programmer, when applicable. Preparing a list of authors, as well as the listed order of authors, before beginning to write will help ensure that all individuals involved in the research study understand at the outset whether they can be an author and, if so, what their contribution should be. The principal investigator of the research is generally the person most responsible for the study and therefore, the first author. The ordering of authors should be agreed upon at the outset. Each author should expect to make a substantial contribution to preparation of and/or critical review of the manuscript.

After selecting co-authors and mentors, the first real step in the writing process is to select a target journal. Consider high-ranking professional journals that are known to you and your colleagues and are a match to your research topic. Think about who would read the research report. Who is the target audience? Are they clinicians in a specific specialty? Is there a specialist journal that matches the target audience? Who is the population in the research? Is there a journal that targets the population? If the audience is educators and the population of interest is patients with diabetes, the target journal might be one that focuses on educators, diabetes, or even diabetic educators.

When writing a scholarly manuscript for publication, always select a *peer-reviewed* or *refereed* journal that contains papers that were reviewed by two or more experts in the field before acceptance and publication. Peer-reviewed papers help ensure quality. Readers expect that published papers passed critical review by experts and that results are trustworthy and accurate. To learn if a journal uses peer review, follow these steps: First, go to the journal site home page and read "about the journal," as peer review status is often listed and there may even be a listing of editorial board members. Second, read the author guidelines for the journal, which often state whether papers will go through a peer review process. Finally, when searching through publication databases, such as *Cumulative Index to Nursing and Allied Health Literature* (CINAHL), the search can be limited to peer-reviewed journals.

Open-access journals are those that are available for free to readers, as the authors generally pay to publish their research. Most open-access journals claim to be peer reviewed, but it may be important to review the editorial board to determine the credibility of the review process. Some open-access journals have the same editorial team as their paper journal counterpart, but others, especially those that are only available online (there is no paper journal counterpart), may be "predator" journals that are not known for publishing high-quality research (Hill, 2015). Your reputation as an author may be based on the quality of the journals in which you publish, so beware of predator publications. Use your mentor to guide you through the journal selection process. Open-access journals are listed through the *Directory of Open Access Journals* (DOAJ), an online directory that indexes and provides access to quality open access, peer-reviewed journals. Before taking the next step, find out the publication fee to publish in an open-access journal. Nearly all charge a fee, due upon acceptance of the paper for publication. Fees can range from $400 to over $3,000. It is important to know the expected fee before you submit a paper to an open-access journal. Journals that are not categorized as open-access do not charge a fee for publishing scholarly research.

The final type of journal is an online journal. Many journals have an online feature that may make your paper an online-only publication (your paper, if accepted is only published online). Alternately, your paper may be electronically published (ePub), a feature whereby soon-to-be published papers are available online prior to publication in a paper journal. Papers published in an online journal may be free to readers or there may be a fee to use, based on journal policies.

Once some journals are selected, determine the best fit by obtaining the author guidelines and reviewing each for journal style and expectations. Author guidelines contain detailed information about the types of manuscripts the editor prefers, maximum length of manuscripts, and formatting details. Find author guidelines by simply typing the name of the journal and "author guidelines" into a search engine and retrieve the html or PDF guidelines online.

Writing a Manuscript

Consider the journal audience so that you write in an appropriate style. For example, submission to a research journal, such as *Journal of Nursing Measurement* or *Clinical Nursing Research*, will have readers who are familiar with research terminology. You will not need to explain terms such as "independent variable" or "external validity." If the journal publishes few research papers, readers may not be well informed in research. Descriptions that limit use of technical research terms may increase readers' understanding of important research methods and results.

Organizing and Formatting your Manuscript
Review a few research papers in the target journal to assess the journal's writing style. Organize and format the manuscript so that reviewers see it is a good fit for the journal. Follow the author guidelines and, when no direction is provided, use the formatting of published research papers in the journal as a guide. Some questions to consider when organizing and formatting a research paper are:

- Should an abstract be included?
- What subheadings are used?
- Are articles written in the first or third person (e.g., *I collected data* or *the researcher collected data?*)
- Are tables and figures used?
- How much space is devoted to each section of the article? For example, is a large part of the article devoted to background or a review of literature, or are there only one or two paragraphs for this?

Many papers are limited to 12 to 15 typed, double-spaced pages, not including references, title page, tables or figures. Think carefully how each section of the paper will be organized before putting pen to paper (fingers to keyboard). Many first-time authors write too much background information and limit the details of the research methods, results, and discussion sections. Decide the approximate length of each section before writing. Table 9.4 illustrates one

TABLE 9.4 Organizing Manuscripts

SECTION	LENGTH
Title Page	One page
Introduction	One-half page
Background/theoretical framework	2 Pages
Methodology	2 Pages
Results	4 Pages
Discussion	2 Pages
Conclusions	2 pages
Limitations	One-half page
Implications	2 pages

way to make a quick organizational scheme for a manuscript limited to 12 to 15 pages. You may want to write a traditional outline that lists bullet points of content for each section.

In the introduction section, orient the reader to independent and dependent study variables and study population, and then the purpose of the study. Include enough background or literature review so that readers will understand the significance of your study in relation to previous research. Be sure to be concise as most content from the introduction to the methods section of the paper is three pages or less. Generally, research questions or hypotheses are in the last paragraph of the introduction section, so that readers understand the reason for the study before they begin reading the methods section. Many nursing journals (but generally not medical journals), request documentation of the conceptual or theoretical framework that guided the research. This content usually is part of the introduction.

In the methods section, present important information that readers would need to replicate the study. Details will help readers judge the validity and quality of methodological procedures. Include information such as power analysis for your sample size, measures used to enhance internal and external validity, and reliability and validity of instruments used. At minimum, the methods section should include the study design and institutional review board approval; setting and subjects, including how the sample size was determined; intervention(s) delivered, when applicable; independent and dependent variables and their measurement; data collection methods; and the data analysis plan.

The results section should match the research's specific aims, questions, or hypothesis, even if there were no significant results. Prior to providing research results, describe the sample (subject) characteristics so the reader can understand if the study population matches the target population. Maintain the same ordering of study themes as presented in the methods section and do not introduce new themes. Points presented in Table 9.1 apply here. Do not interpret results in this section; just provide results in a very factual way. Use subheaders or new paragraphs to separate study themes.

The discussion section is intended to show how your results relate to those of other research studies, as well as to describe study limitations and implications for clinical practice and future research. Be sure to reference the literature in this section. Only discuss topics related to your study. Also, be careful not to simply reword the results. Discuss your results and provide a one-paragraph conclusion at the end. The conclusion should not introduce new content or have references.

Once a first draft of the manuscript is complete, it is time to think about revisions. It is typical to have multiple drafts before submission to the journal. More drafts mean a higher quality submission since it is likely that errors will be corrected in every revision. Read the manuscript carefully to ensure alignment exists among the research questions/hypotheses, methodology, results, and discussion. Find a few colleagues or friends who are not familiar with the research study and ask them to read and critique the manuscript. Ask for honest feedback regarding clarity of each section, formatting issues, and suggestions for strengthening the quality of the paper. Make all revisions, read the manuscript again, and check it with each requirement of the author guidelines to make sure all requirements for the journal are met. Check all references for accuracy and proper formatting. Review for redundancy of wording, excess wording ("also," "the," "very," "however," "thus," and "additionally" are common), proper tense (e.g., review of literature and results are written in past tense), and consistency in word choices (e.g., if you choose the wording "clinical nurses" [versus "staff nurses"], use "clinical nurses" consistently throughout the paper). In another re-read, ensure that wording structure uses active voice. Then, once ready, send to all co-authors to review and sign-off. The statistician should carefully review all tables and figures for accuracy, the data analysis plan in the methods section, and the results section of the manuscript. Validate that URL links are still current for accessing online documents.

Submitting the Manuscript

Author guidelines will include specific information about manuscript submittal to the target journal. Nearly all manuscripts are submitted electronically and may require the first author to register prior to paper submission. It is common that manuscript sections are uploaded separately, for example, the title page, and each table and figure are separate documents from the sections that contain the abstract, manuscript text, and references. Some journals require a cover letter. If requested, write a brief (one page) cover letter that states why you feel the manuscript is appropriate for the journal and why you are an appropriate first author of the manuscript. Some general rules about writing a cover letter are: address it to the editor by name; state the date; and use three short paragraphs: one to introduce the paper title, the second to provide rationale why it should be published, and the third to provide disclosures, funding sources, or other information the editor should know about.

Submit the manuscript to only one journal. It is unethical to send a manuscript to more than one journal while it is actively in review. If the review process is too long, you must write a letter to the editor asking for permission to rescind the paper before submitting to another journal.

Behind the Scenes After Manuscript Submission

Within 1 to 2 weeks, the first author should expect to receive an e-mail from the editor or managing editor that the manuscript was received by the journal. At this time, or by separate e-mail, the first author will also receive a manuscript number that may be different from the submission number. Do not lose the manuscript number as all further correspondence with the journal editor may require that number. Receiving a manuscript number is usually a sign that the paper is being assigned to reviewers. If you do not receive confirmation that the manuscript was received, first, go to the submittal system to be sure you submitted the paper correctly. If you did, check the junk or spam folder of your Internet mailbox. If no correspondence was found, contact the editor.

After confirmation of manuscript submission, you may have a short or long wait to receive peer-review feedback. Most manuscripts are assigned to two or three reviewers, and they may be given 1 to 2 months to provide written feedback on the manuscript. A long wait period could be due to reviewers agreeing to review but failing to follow through, extra reviews requested if feedback is wildly divergent among reviewers, or a request for statistical review.

Once all reviewers have completed reviews and submitted them to the journal editor, the editor will write a decision letter about acceptability of the manuscript for publication. There are three common decisions: One—and the most exciting!—is that the manuscript was accepted for publication in its present form. This outcome only occurs about 2% of the time, so do not expect this response. The second decision is a rejection. This outcome is discouraging but it does not always mean that the manuscript was not important or was poorly written. Sometimes the editor believes that the manuscript is a low priority based on readership needs or that the manuscript is not the best match for the journal. Rejection rates vary by journal. Some critically acclaimed journals have a 70% to 80% rejection rate, as they simply receive too many submissions and only accept those that they feel are the most novel, will get the greatest press, or have the biggest impact on moving health science forward. Also, editors may reject a paper that has poor formatting or sentence structure, even if the theme is novel and the research methods are high quality.

The third type of decision is that the paper requires minor or major revisions, then resubmission for reconsideration for publication. This is a more common outcome of manuscript submission. If you receive a request for revision and resubmission, you should cautiously celebrate. Although resubmission does not guarantee acceptance, if all reviewer requests are addressed adequately and correctly, there is a strong possibility it will be eventually accepted, pending revisions that match reviewers' requests.

Reviewers will likely be anonymous to you, but their comments should form the basis of the revisions made. Reviewers want your paper to be high quality so that readers can trust your results and replicate or translate your work. Their role is to provide constructive feedback to improve the paper. Occasionally, comments may seem harsh. Do not misinterpret the criticism as a personal attack; remember, reviewers want a high-quality paper and their comments are meant to help you strengthen the manuscript. Read all comments, set them aside for a few days, and then read them again. Share reviewer feedback with your writing mentor and co-authors and develop revisions together. Before resubmitting, have an expert writer provide feedback to you. If reviewers commented on writing style, formatting, or sentence structure, a review by a seasoned author or editor may uncover further revisions needed.

If the requests for revision are major, and would change the substance of the manuscript, an alternate option is to rescind the paper and submit the manuscript to another journal. However, there is a risk that the new journal editor may send the paper to the same reviewer(s). If that happens and no revisions were made, there is a high likelihood the paper will be rejected. Also,

TABLE 9.5 Response to Request for Manuscript Revisions

REVIEWER #1	AUTHOR'S RESPONSES
1. It was a nice read. Adding content in areas provided more depth and clarity on this topic.	Thank you for the kind remarks.
2. The implementation section: The focus is on research hospital organizations. Later on (no page numbers) in the Practicality and Reusability of *** the manuscript refers to the "education academic setting in which teaching, research and scholarship are integral. . . ." However, in the implementation section only research and monies are mentioned. All three are integral in the success of an academic career—it is important to discuss all three in the beginning of the paper so the later section connects it all.	I have added the following two sentences (page 1, Implementation section, last two sentences): "Last, teaching is a part of most academic workloads. Faculty candidates need to know what courses they might be expected to teach and have academic preparation related to teaching and learning."
3. Monies—maybe use grant funding in support of research and sustaining research and scholarship.	This change has been made. The sentence (page 1, Implementation section, sentence 4) now reads: "Most research-intensive universities are looking for faculty candidates who can not only advance the science of nursing, but also bring grant funding into the school to support the research and the researcher's salary."
4. Was permission granted in the filming and evaluation portion of the project?	Yes.
REVIEWER #2	AUTHOR'S RESPONSES
1. The limitations section—I would add this was more than a convenience sample; these were attendees at a simulation conference. This would not necessarily represent the general nursing education population using simulation. The participants also self-selected and presented themselves to the booth. Important to recognize this limitation and recommend repeating (as you did). You may find more schools are in the early stages of Rogers's theory.	Thank you for this great suggestion. We have added a Limitations section to be more transparent. We have also included the word "targeted" before "convenience sample" to better indicate that it was more than a typical convenience sample.

starting with another journal can lengthen the time of peer review and prolong publication. Thus, it is often recommended to make the requested revisions and resubmit to the original journal.

Part of the revision process includes clear communication to the editor about responses to each request for revision, even if the consensus was not to make changes. Provide rationale to the editor and reviewers. Table 9.5 illustrates one format that can be used to communicate revisions to the editor and reviewers. Itemized responses to each requested change or comment should be clearly written and reflect an understanding of the revision request. Authors should understand that most likely, the revised manuscript and response to the editor and reviewers will be sent to the original reviewers, who will know if the authors failed to make requested changes or if changes remain inadequate.

VOICE OF A NURSE RESEARCHER

Cynthia Bautista, PhD, RN, CNRN, SCRN, CCNS, ACNS-BC, FNCS
Neuroscience Clinical Nurse Specialist, Yale–New Haven Hospital,
New Haven, Connecticut

I was asked to coordinate the first poster session at our hospital's Nursing Research Day. Two colleagues and I met to create the call for poster abstracts. We first reviewed other organizations' calls for poster abstracts so we could create something very informative. Once the call was disseminated, we began to create our poster abstract score card. This score card was based on objectives from the research conference and similar criteria seen at other organizations' poster abstract reviews. As the poster abstracts began to filter in, we met to grade the submissions based on the criteria we had decided upon. We first graded them individually and then met as a group to discuss our results. Once we had agreed on the poster presenters, we then sent out acceptance letters with all the information to display their posters at the nursing research conference.

I have given a couple of podium presentations on the various research studies I participated in. Lessons I learned were (a) to watch someone else present their study. I was able to pick up many helpful hints in the presentation. Once I had created my presentation, (b) to practice, practice, practice, paying attention to timing. Many times you are only given about 20 minutes to present your

(*continued*)

> ## VOICE OF A NURSE RESEARCHER (*continued*)
>
> research. (c) Have a colleague listen to your presentation and give you feedback. The day of the presentation, (d) bring copies of articles previously reviewed and data collection tools to share with the audience. Finally, (e) have business cards available to pass out at the end of the presentation in case someone is interested in collaborating on another research study.
>
> For publication in a peer-reviewed journal, my experiences were with a group of colleagues. The first thing to decide is whose name goes first, second, and last. Be sure to learn the ordering of authors up front. Next, expect to be assigned or assign yourself sections of the manuscript to write. When everyone takes a section, it is not so overwhelming. One person tends to facilitate the group and will put all the sections together as they are written. Expect to be asked to read the entire manuscript to see if it flows, and to make edits where needed. Once manuscripts are submitted, I anxiously wait for the editor and manuscript reviewers responses. Most of the time, there are many revisions to make, with lots of excellent suggestions to strengthen our written words. After making revisions as suggested, and resubmitting, we wait hopefully for editor acceptance of the paper for publication. It is a great feeling to see your hard work in print.

SUMMARY

Research is incomplete until results are disseminated. Disseminating results, whether internally or externally, by media, poster, oral presentation, or publication, requires effort and attention to detail. The outcome is usually personally and professionally satisfying; research results, once disseminated, may lead to new research and clinical practice changes that close the research-to-practice gap and improve clinical outcomes.

REFERENCES

DeSilets, L. D. (2010). Poster presentations. *The Journal of Continuing Education in Nursing, 41*(10), 437–438.

DeVan, M., & Baum, N. (2013). Public speaking: Creating presentations that are awe inspiring not yawn producing. *Journal of Medical Practice Management, 29*(3), 204–205.

Directory of Open Access Journals (DOAJ). Retrieved at http://doaj.org/

Durkin, G. (2011). Promoting professional development through poster presentations. *Journal for Nurses in Staff Development, 27*(3), E1-3.

Hill, K. S. (2015). Predatory publishing: What nurse executives need to know. *JONA, 45*(2), 59–60.

Ilic, D., & Rowe, N. (2013). What is the evidence that poster presentations are effective in promoting knowledge transfer? A state of the art review. *Health Information and Libraries Journal, 30*, 4–12.

Greenhalgh, T., de Jongste, J. C., & Brand, P. L. P. (2011). Preparing and delivering a 10-minute presentation at a scientific meeting. *Pediatric Respiratory Review, 12*, 148–149. doi: 10.1016/j.prrv.2011.01.010

Hoffman, M., & Mittelman, M. (2004). Presentations at professional meetings: Notes, suggestions and tips for speakers. *European Journal of Internal Medicine, 15*, 358–363.

Longo, A., & Tierney, C. (2012). Presentation skills for the nurse educator. *Journal for Nurses in Staff Development, 28*(1), 16–23. doi: 10.1097./NND.0b013e318240a699

McClendon, K. S., & Stover, K. R. (2014). Tips for a successful poster presentation. *American Journal of Health-System Pharmacy, 71*, 449–451.

Yang, J. (2010). Mastering the big talk: Preparing an oral presentation. *Gastrointestinal Endocscopy, 71*(7), 1275–1276.

Nancy M. Albert
Sandra L. Siedlecki

10

EVALUATING YOUR NURSING RESEARCH PROGRAM AND NURTURING IT FOR LONG-TERM SUCCESS

EVALUATING YOUR NURSING RESEARCH PROGRAM

Research program success can take on many forms and will most likely be based on the vision, mission, and values of your hospital organization and nursing department. To be successful, a *vertical infrastructure* of resources must be available, so that all nurses have access to formal support structures to navigate and facilitate the research experience (see Chapters 2 and 3). However, the infrastructure needs to be coupled with context related to embedding research into the fabric of hospital nursing at every level (*horizontal infrastructure*). Highest-level nursing leadership must ask those who report to them what they have done in the last year to advance nursing science and to ensure nursing practices are evidence based. Nurse managers at the unit level must also consider how their nursing teams are ensuring that care planning and delivery are evidence based. Nurse managers must assess their teams' priorities to ensure they are considering what they have done to create new nursing knowledge, and how they have aided in the process of advancing new knowledge published by others. Chapter 7 provides some examples of horizontal structure, most notably, embedding nursing research in a clinical/career ladder at *every* level and having a "model" of evidence-based nursing practice that encourages clinical nurses to question and explore current nursing practices and take action when ideas for interventions are raised or when nursing research questions are developed. Translation of nursing research can be a slow process (see Chapter 8), but it is important to act on best practices that will impact clinical and administrative outcomes, and it should be part of a "research evaluation" assessment.

HOW WILL WE KNOW WHAT WORKS FOR
OUR HOSPITAL ORGANIZATION?

The depth and breadth of research infrastructure needed to be successful will depend on many factors, such as size of the hospital and external nursing research resources directly available to the nursing team. Hospitals that have formal academic–clinical contracted relationships with colleges of nursing may not need to spend time developing and nurturing some vertical infrastructures, as resources may be available through the college; however, regular assessment is warranted, as seemingly ideal academic–clinical relationships on paper may not parlay into research outcomes or even meet research process needs of clinicians who seek research services. Likewise, and maybe even more important, horizontal structures must be regularly assessed and updated to ensure that nurse clinicians have opportunities to initiate and complete nursing research projects, and disseminate and translate new knowledge globally.

Assessing Research Outcomes

Annually, when nursing leadership goals and strategies are assessed, nursing research should be reviewed. First, where does nursing research "fit" within nursing organization goals? Within the Nursing Institute at the Cleveland Clinic, research goals are formally placed under the global theme "impact" as nursing research can create many impacts, such as (a) branding the department as leaders of high-quality nursing care, (b) creating revenue streams through innovations and inventions, (c) ensuring clinical practice matches highest evidence-based practice, safety and quality standards, and clinical outcomes, and (d) promoting professional clinical nurse development. Figure 10.1 depicts direct and indirect relationships between nursing research and nursing excellence and Figure 10.2 depicts how leading nursing research as a lived experience (not just something others do) can create revenue; decrease spending; aid in purchasing (supplies and equipment), process, and informatics decisions; and, ultimately, promote nursing excellence. Some examples based on nursing research from the Cleveland Clinic exemplify principles from the figures.

- Prior to the economic recession of 2007 to 2009, there was a trend toward using disposables, rather than reusable products in patient care. As pressure to improve quality by decreasing hospital-acquired infections accelerated, companies began marketing disposable products as a means to decrease hospital-acquired infections (as part of a bundled intervention or as a single intervention). One such item was electrocardiographic (ECG) lead wires used to monitor intensive care and telemetry patients. Our first step

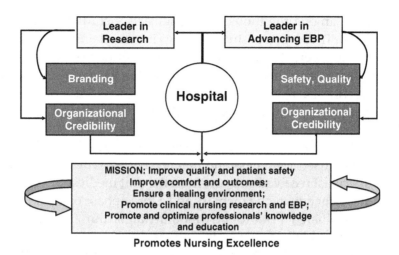

FIGURE 10.1 Nursing Research Promotes Nursing Excellence.
EBP, evidence based practices.

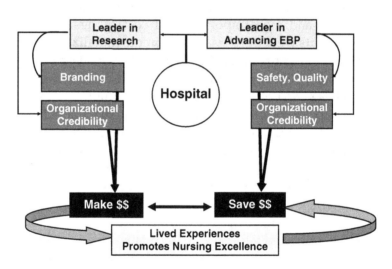

FIGURE 10.2 Leading Nursing Research, as a Lived Experience, Promotes Fiscal Responsibility.

in research was to learn what types of bacteria and fungus grew on reusable ECG lead wires (Albert et al., 2010). Once we learned that bacteria were present on cleaned, ready-to-use ECG lead wires, the next phase of research was to learn if reusable lead wires were a culprit in hospital-acquired infections. To answer a "cause–effect" question, a randomized, controlled research design was needed. We conducted the research among multiple paired medical, surgical, cardiothoracic, and neurological intensive care units, and much to the surprise of the company whose disposable ECG lead wires were used and our own nurse managers, there were no differences in infection rates among the thousands of subjects included in the trial (Albert et al., 2014). Translation of study findings meant retaining reusable ECG lead wires, as they were durable, and the systems and supplies used in cleaning were much less expensive than the cost of purchasing disposable ECG lead wires.

- In critical care, early mobilization of patients became more prevalent in the research literature after 2009; however, in neurological critical care settings, health care providers were reluctant to advocate for early mobility as patients had intracranial catheters that were tenuously placed, and disorders that caused weakness and balance issues. Our neurological clinical nurse specialist received support from the unit medical director to create an algorithm for advancing mobility and a three-phase comparative research project was initiated. Prior to early mobility algorithm/intervention, most patients remained in bed during their intensive care stay (Mulkey, Bena, & Albert, 2014); however, in both early (4 month) and late (10 month) postintervention assessment, early mobility increased (Klein, Mulkey, Bena, & Albert, 2015). In addition, there were no adverse events, some quality metrics improved, and there was a large, clinically (and statistically) significant reduction in unit and hospital length of stay postintervention compared to preintervention. Sharing results internally led to continued implementation of early mobility and, more important, with cost savings from earlier discharge, new ceiling lifts were purchased to promote mobilization efforts.

- A director of nursing quality hypothesized that predictors of hospital-based fall events differed among cancer and noncancer patients. Her hypothesis was based on noticing younger ages and higher rates of blood transfusions and pain medication among cancer patients who fell compared to patients with other medical–surgical diagnoses. To test her hypothesis, a descriptive research study was completed to examine characteristics of cancer patients who fell. Authors compared the characteristics identified with published research on the general population of hospitalized patients who fell (Capone, Albert, Bena, & Morrison, 2010). After learning that there were some similar and dissimilar factors, a comparative study was initiated to learn if specific factors predicted fall events in hospitalized patients being treated for cancer. Of more than 20 factors that were identified in the descriptive report, seven factors predicted falls, and all but two were fairly unique to patients with cancer (Capone, Albert, Bena, & Tang, 2012). More recently, a validation study was led by a clinical nurse working in the inpatient palliative care unit. The goals were to determine if the seven predictors of falls remained important in a new cohort of patients with cancer, and if the fall event predictors were more important than the six-factor Morse fall assessment tool (usual care). After sharing results with the cancer leadership team, the new falls tool was implemented in a hospital-based palliative care unit, and the nursing director recently reported that the unit had a 50-day span without a single fall event. Informatics technology personnel created an electronic reporting system to enhance widespread use of the tool, and plans are in place to use the tool in all hospital units that focus on cancer care. To support the costs of research, the tool was made available for use by other hospitals for a small fee.

- Clinical nurses working on a nutrition support team (parenteral nutrition through peripherally inserted central catheters or Hickman catheters) wondered if the risk of postdischarge catheter-based infection and other complications could be reduced. Nurses and nutrition therapy personnel collaborated to develop a randomized, controlled research study to examine if patients who received usual care education during hospitalization (verbal and written materials about maintenance and care of catheter and dressing) or usual care plus an educational intervention (posthospital discharge education reinforcement via a voice-over PowerPoint digital video device therapy) had better clinical outcomes. There were no differences in catheter-related bloodstream infections or rehospitalization between groups (Emery, Pearson, Lopez, Hamilton, & Albert, 2015). Knowing that usual care in hospital education and written materials were adequate in preventing complications was an important finding, as it allowed nurses to focus on other areas of need.

- Medical intensive care and medical unit patients tend to be elderly and may require fecal management systems. Intensive care nurses believed that 40% of patients developed anal erosions from fecal management systems. Further, when the product evaluation committee made a decision to switch fecal management system products, intensive care nurses verbalized their beliefs that the new system was inferior (based on product features) and that anal erosions would increase. No literature was found on the rate of anal erosions from fecal management systems. Rather than making product decisions based on emotion and past preferences, a randomized, controlled research study was developed and partially funded by one of the companies that produce fecal management systems. Nurses learned that the anal erosion rate was much lower than their self-assessment and that there were no differences in anal erosion rates between products (Sammon et al., 2015). The research findings increased nurses' insight about true anal erosion rates and that lower cost products were not necessarily inferior, merely based on features.

These five examples provide a glimpse of outcomes achieved that led to translation of new knowledge in clinical practice, prevention of unnecessary spending, wise purchasing of equipment and products, and translation of new knowledge through validation research, followed by implementation of the new assessment methodology. By generating research findings, nurses can streamline practices and make cost- and time-effective decisions.

Before research outcomes can inform clinical practice decisions, the research design and methods need to be rigorous. Rigorous research includes a sample size based on review of the literature, use of valid and reliable measures, and an analysis that controls for moderating factors. When possible, multicenter (or at least multi-unit) hospital-based studies are preferred as findings are more generalizable. When considering what works for a hospital organization, it will be important for nursing and nurse researcher leaders to be able to differentiate high- from low-quality research findings, so that decisions about translating findings into practice are made with an understanding of study limitations and biases. Finally, nurse researchers need to understand outcome expectations set by leadership. If nursing leaders do not understand differences between high- and low-quality research and want research to inform clinical practice—not just be an exercise that meets a need for clinician-led nursing research—then it is up to nurse researchers to ensure resources support high-quality research.

Evaluating Research Structures, Processes, and Systems

Research outcomes are interwoven with research structures, processes, and systems, since the robustness of available research processes and systems can impact outcomes. Thus, nurse researchers will need to regularly evaluate factors that generate desired research outcomes. If a nursing research department or nursing unit leaders have great success in getting clinical nurses excited about research, but at the end of the year, research outcomes are lacking, goals and structures may need to be updated. Examples of global targets that indicate a need to evaluate a research program are:

- Less than 2.5% of all nurse employees are involved in nursing research projects
- Less than one active (institutional review board [IRB] approved) research project per 100 hospital beds
- An excessive number of stagnant and abandoned projects

All three scenarios, individually or in combination, reduce the ability to produce new knowledge that informs clinical practices. Although it may be difficult to determine the exact elements of success or failure of a nursing research program, it is important to consider a continuous improvement strategy to ensure that the right combination of structures, processes, and systems are present and that challenges to success are addressed. Finally, as described in Chapter 2, doctorate-prepared nurse researchers in our hospital organization must meet annual performance expectations to achieve a "fully meets" performance rating and participate in a mentor/coach–mentee evaluation process. Written performance expectations ensure that team members are productive and are meeting clinical nurses' needs. Further, their success in meeting performance expectations leads to nursing department success.

NURTURING A NURSING RESEARCH PROGRAM FOR LONG-TERM SUCCESS

Long-term success and sustainability over time are important goals for a nursing research program. The success of an established program provides additional benefits and an opportunity to spread your influence as a generator of nursing knowledge. Some benefits include collaborative opportunities with academic institutions, other health care organizations, and other disciplines. Collaborative opportunities provide access to larger populations for studies, which in turn improve generalizability of study findings.

Partnering With Academic Institutions

An established nursing research program in a health care organization is the ideal partner for nurses in academic institutions interested in conducting clinical research but need a partner who has access to patient populations. Each collaborative partnership needs to be structured in a way that provides advantages for both the nurse faculty in the academic institution and the doctorate-prepared nurse researchers in the health care organization. It is important that agreements include intellectual property rights, including authorship of all manuscripts submitted and grant dollars when funded.

Partnering With Other Health Care Organizations

Established nursing research programs are attractive to health care organizations interested in participating in nursing research, but lacking internal resources to accomplish this alone. Partnerships are advantageous to both health care organizations. They provide access to larger and more diverse populations that allow greater generalizability of findings for the established research department, and they provide the partnering facilities the opportunity to learn about the research process through their access to experienced nurse researchers and other available resources. As with academic partnerships, it is important that agreements about intellectual property rights be agreed upon prior to any joint projects.

Partnering With Other Disciplines

Because nursing and nursing care are not delivered in a vacuum, and many disciplines are involved in patient outcomes, it is critical to think of how other disciplines can be included in research projects. Useful collaborations may be with physicians, pharmacists, nutritionists, or any other discipline appropriate to a study. Since resources for research are most likely supported primarily by the nursing research department budget, a nurse should be the principal investigator and initiator of interdisciplinary studies. Again, as with other collaborations, it is important that agreements about intellectual property rights and authorship be established prior to the start of each project.

SUCCESS BREEDS SUCCESS

The Impact of Dissemination

The hallmark of a mature and established nursing research program is its sphere of influence. Influence is not a result of conducting nursing research, but of the dissemination of nursing research findings to the larger national and international nursing community, and to the health care community in general. Nurse researchers are a major resource for nurses who completed their research studies and are ready to disseminate their findings. Methods of dissemination can be poster and oral presentations at national and international conferences. However, the true measure of an established program is the number of research studies published in high-quality peer-reviewed literature.

The Impact of a Nursing Research Conference

The final hallmark of a mature and established nursing research program is the ability to sponsor a research conference that brings in nurses from all over the country and all over the world. The idea is to not only showcase your organization's research, but to provide nurses interested in conducting nursing research an opportunity to network with and discuss opportunities with other nurses who are conducting research. Initially a conference is a costly undertaking. However as the reputation of the nursing research department grows, so does that of the conference. The goal is to eventually have a self-sustaining conference that pays for itself through conference registration fees.

Attracting Attendees
Advance planning (a year in advance) and advertising through professional websites, word-of-mouth from hospital colleagues, and e-mail lists to nurses in academia and professional organizations are essential to the success of any conference. It is important to have an agenda and speakers that will attract nurses from outside your organization. Also, the location needs to be considered. Finding a location that provides attendees with a good experience (at the conference and also in the surrounding community) will help to promote

future conference attendance. The more professional and successful your conference is, the more your sphere of influence will grow. A quality conference will attract repeat attendees. Providing an opportunity for poster and oral presentations through a call for abstracts is another way to attract nurses to the conference. Typically, it is customary to offer poster and oral presenters a registration discount. A discount can be extended to both the primary author and one or two additional authors of collaborative projects. A reduction in registration costs may actually encourage more people to attend.

Funding a Conference

Initially a nursing research conference will require internal funding. However, once established, registration fees will provide much, if not all, of the financial support required. In addition, the Agency for Healthcare Research and Quality (AHRQ) offers two conference grants to support professional conferences. The small conference grant is available at a maximum of $35,000 and a large conference grant is available at a maximum of $100,000. These conference grants are competitive, with only a few awarded each year. However, grant writing is a skill that nurse researchers possess and writing this grant can be a joint writing project for the nurse researcher team. When considering this type of grant support, it is important to remember that these funds cannot be used for honoraria, food, or conference giveaways with the organization's logo on it. However, it can be used for site rental, audio-visual costs for personnel and equipment, and costs associated with speakers (speaker fees and travel costs).

CONCLUSION

Although there are growing pains and costs associated with the formation of a nursing research department, the eventual benefits enhance the nursing department and hospital organization's image. Being known as a health care organization that is a leader in both the use and generation of nursing knowledge has its own benefits in terms of nursing research opportunities.

REFERENCES

Albert, N. M., Hancock, K., Murray, T., Karafa, M., Runner, J. C., Fowler, S. B., . . . Krajewski, S. (2010). Cleaned, ready-to-use, reusable electrocardiographic lead wires as a source of pathogenic microorganisms. *American Journal of Critical Care, 19*:e73–80. doi: 10.4037/ajcc2010304

Albert, N. M., Slifcak, E., Roach, J. D., Bena, J. F., Horvath, G., Wilson, S., . . . Murray, T. (2014). Infection rates in intensive care units by electrocardiographic lead wire type: Disposable vs. reusable. *American Journal of Critical Care, 23*, 460–467. doi: 10.4037/ajcc2014362

Capone, L. J., Albert, N. M., Bena, J. F., & Morrison, S. M. (2010). Characteristics of hospitalized cancer patients who fall. *Journal of Nursing Care Quality, 25*, 216–223. doi: 10.1097/NCQ.0b013e3181d4a1ce

Capone, L. J., Albert, N. M., Bena, J. F., & Tang, A. S. (2012). Predictors of a fall event in hospitalized patients with cancer. *Oncology Nursing Forum, 39*, E407–15. doi: 10.1188/12.ONF.E407–E415

Emery, D., Pearson, A., Lopez, R., Hamilton, C., & Albert, N. M. (2015). Voiceover interactive PowerPoint catheter care education for home parenteral nutrition. *Nutrition in Clinical Practice, 30*, 714–719. doi: 10.1177/0884533615584391

Klein, K., Mulkey, M., Bena, J. F., & Albert, N. M. (2015). Clinical and psychological effects of early mobilization in patients treated in a neurologic ICU: A comparative study. *Critical Care Medicine, 43*, 865–873. doi: 10.1097/CCM.0000000000000787

Mulkey, M., Bena, J. F., & Albert, N. M. (2014). Clinical outcomes of patient mobility in a neuroscience intensive care unit. *Journal of Neuroscience Nursing, 46*, 153–161. doi: 10.1097/JNN.0000000000000053

Sammon, M. A., Montague, M., Frame, F., Guzman, D., Bena, J. F., Palascak, A., & Albert, N. M. (2015). Randomized controlled study of the effects of 2 fecal management systems on incidence of anal erosion. *Journal of Wound Ostomy Continence Nursing, 42*, 279–286. doi: 10.1097/WON.0000000000000128

Jayne S. Rosenberger
Susan J. McCrudden
Mary Beth Modic

11

LESSONS LEARNED FROM
NURSES CONDUCTING RESEARCH

EDITOR'S NOTE

This chapter provides two stories of lessons learned. The first section, "Improving Medical–Surgical Practices," provides lessons learned from clinically based novice nurse researchers. The second section, "Stories from the Field," is by a clinical nurse specialist research investigator. Both stories provide unique perspectives and "lessons learned" that may stimulate and/or help sustain a culture of inquiry and nursing research.

IMPROVING MEDICAL–SURGICAL PRACTICES

Jayne S. Rosenberger and Susan J. McCrudden

This section of the chapter is a reflection of nursing research conducted by two clinical nurses (hereafter labeled as Jayne and Susan), who float among hospital units based on staffing needs. We each have more than 33 years of nursing experience; however, the combined years of research experience before embarking on our current research studies was zero. We are novice research nurses who are writing about our first research projects. It is our hope that the experiences and lessons learned from our stories will resonate with other nurses, and that readers will sense our newly found passion for advancing nursing science to promote the highest level of clinical nursing practices. Stories are related to how our research studies were born and developed into study proposals and institutional review board (IRB) applications; our adventures in tool use, data collection, and data cleaning; how we came to understand analysis reports; and the value of mentorship.

BEGINNINGS OF TWO RESEARCH STUDIES

Developing Research Questions

The first research question was developed after I (Jayne) attended a 3-hour "research overview workshop" that focused on helping clinical nurses recognize the importance of research and how to get started. The doctorate-prepared nurse researcher who led the class discussed using the PICO (patient population, intervention, comparative group, and outcome) framework to develop a research question. To demonstrate how to develop a PICO question, she presented a slide of four bottles of pills and asked participants to develop a PICO question based on the visual picture. My first thought was how prescription bottles looked (the same shape, coloring, caps, and label) and wondered how patients could tell one medication from another, especially if they had health literacy, sight, or other limitations. As part of the research workshop I went to the library and conducted a literature review on the topic: color-coded prescription bottles. The literature review produced multiple research papers on medication adherence, but very little was found on helping patients understand how to identify prescription bottle contents as unique medications. I reported the literature review findings to the group and members provided advice about alternative research questions and outcomes. Participants explored how to color code bottles so each was unique. The ideas of colored dots or caps were discussed. At the end of the research overview workshop, I solidified the research question and the methodology plan, which was to be an interventional research study to determine if a system of color coding medication bottles was effective in increasing patient's medication adherence.

Lesson 1: There is ample support to move a research idea forward within our hospital, even if the initial idea seems daunting and complex.

For a second research study that we (Jayne and Susan) jointly developed, involvement began without any thought of research. As background, float nurses are used to being flexible in meeting the policies and procedures of each unit in which they work. At a shared governance council meeting, team members discussed that in the coronary care unit (CCU), nurses obtained blood pressures (BPs) in both arms, but in other intensive care units (ICUs), BPs were only obtained in one arm on admission. After being intrigued by unit differences, we looked for answers that would explain the rationale and value of inter-arm versus single-arm BPs at unit admission. A critical care clinical nurse specialist provided assistance by sharing an American Association of Critical-Care Nurses (AACN) practice alert on obtaining BPs at ICU admission. References in the alert were more than 5 years old and the level of evidence was D, reflecting expert opinion; thus, the next step was to conduct a new review of the literature. Research-based papers were found, but we needed assistance in interpreting the research results of each paper and also in determining the strength and quality of individual research studies and systematic reviews/meta analyses. A doctorate-prepared nurse researcher was consulted. In a joint review, we learned that the research literature focused on ambulatory and acute care populations and did not address the ICU population. She suggested we initiate a research project to learn the significance of obtaining inter-arm BPs at ICU admission.

> *Lesson 2*: A good mentor can spot a research opportunity after synthesizing the literature and discussing findings.

As novice research nurses who had initiated the medication adherence study (discussed previously), there was doubt that nursing leadership would support us, the same two nurses, to lead the start up of a second research study. We approached our direct supervisor, who was supportive of our involvement in a second project. The nurse researcher suggested that ICU nurses and nurse leaders gather for an informational meeting, which she agreed to attend to lend support. The goal was to determine interest and support for initiating research that would involve clinical nurses. At the meeting, the results of a meta-analysis and the AACN practice alert were reviewed. Five PICO questions were developed and a new research study was born. We were happy that those present for the informational meeting were very positive and encouraging. Their responses created excitement and facilitated our forming a research team. Interestingly enough, the research team was composed of nurses who were not present at the informational gathering, aside from us; however, the robust response showed nurse excitement in being involved in clinical, bedside research. At our hospital, research was moving from being a boring term to one that created new opportunity to get answers to questions and address clinical practice.

Since there were multiple nurses involved in our research project, we learned the necessity of advance meeting planning. Meeting dates were prescheduled via group consensus. The principal investigator (Jayne) recognized the value of having a reliable confidant and supporter (Susan) who had a high level of commitment to the project. Susan was designated the study coordinator to ensure smooth operations in the event of Jayne's absence and to increase availability of key study personnel who could discuss data collection issues and problem solve.

> *Lesson 3*: Having a strong core team is essential to successfully implementing (conducting) a research study that requires clinical nurse support.

Although we had support from the study team, the level of commitment varied by individual nurses. Two team members dropped out due to inability to meet time commitments, one early in the proposal-writing stage, due to family obligations, and the other right before study startup, which neither of us anticipated. The loss of two team members, who were coworkers, was not only stressful, but also was a disappointment for the group. The remaining team members absorbed the additional work and maintained a positive outlook. The value of commitment to research, in terms of both time and intellectual property, was heightened after losing team members. Jayne sent Susan a note of appreciation for consistent meeting attendance, especially since meetings involved work shifts, and poor attendance at scheduled meetings increased the level of responsibility for the entire study team.

> *Lesson 4*: Not all co-investigators are created equal in their commitment to research, allocation of time to research, and in working assertively to meet research goals/milestones.

Proposal Development

Clinical nurse support and technology were factors that affected the proposal development process. Proposal development varied in the two research studies, although they were both quantitative designs. Subjects, study themes, settings, and co-investigators differed, creating diverse energies among the two research study teams. The overall research experience expanded our role as clinical nurses, and inspired us to believe we could have a positive impact on our profession. After recognizing that our patients had difficulty with medication adherence, it was refreshing and exciting to be able to provide a possible solution. However, the research study was not always met with equal enthusiasm. We were asked why we were conducting this research. Susan's response that "it's a problem" did not resonate with clinical nurses in the outpatient setting. In hindsight, we recognized that the answer was direct and simple, but clinical nurses had not previously been able to be advocates for impacting patient care. Although change is common in hospital organizations, involvement in change was not a comfortable fit for some nurses; they had to stretch their previous boundaries to contribute to proposal development. Thus, during this phase of the medication adherence study, we relied heavily on our nurse researcher mentor. Templates from our research website were used as a framework to begin the writing process. Team members used phone conferences with nurse researcher mentors to keep the writing momentum moving forward, and we learned to compile questions in advance so we were prepared to discuss specific topics at meetings.

> *Lesson 5*: Cooperation and support from clinical nurses differs based on history of role autonomy, which is reflected in an ability for clinical, nonmanagerial nurses to discuss problems and create solutions to improve workplace experiences, and for clinical nurses, rather than physicians, to develop systems and processes that may improve patient care and enhance patient adherence to the plan of care.

We quickly realized that we were out of practice with writing, which presented a challenge. We found that computer programs (e.g., using Microsoft Word software) presented a myriad of unanticipated hurdles. We learned the value of routinely saving our work, after losing an entire session of the proposal. Clinical nurses do not require Word document skills to provide patient care, but do for proposal writing. It took time to decrease our dependence on technological support, and we have still not mastered how to use many program features.

We also learned that computers and conference rooms were not created equal. It was impossible to combine time in a clinical setting with time spent in developing the research proposal, even if time was available for research when in a clinical unit, because electronic access to research files was not available at bedside or work station computers. Computers in the library and conference rooms were set up with personal sign-on access, allowing us to use and store our research work on the shared drive. Technological obstacles encountered throughout the proposal development process included conference room equipment that was not in working order; printers located in close proximity to conference rooms that were not associated with the conference room computer, preventing an ability to print work; and computers that were not uniformly equipped with the same software or software versions. Conference rooms are selected based on availability, without knowledge of specific software capabilities that may be required to complete tasks scheduled at the meeting. For example, not all computers had full Microsoft Office programs installed, such as Publisher. Lack of uniformity of computer resources created inefficiency of time, even though we were very cost conscious of optimal use of time and wanted to use this resource in a responsible way.

> *Lesson 6*: Look (and act) before you leap, in terms of ensuring the right resources are available at the right time and that at least one member of the writing team is proficient in technological skills, so that meeting goals are met.

Despite our shortcomings, the nursing research mentors for each research study were always supportive and patient. We were directed to resources for referencing format, which was available in our hospital library. Communication between Susan and me (Jayne) was not always convenient, since our clinical schedules were asynchronous and we often floated to different units when working the same days. It became necessary to communicate through our work e-mail system to connect with co-investigators, mentors, and leadership. We learned that we were not adept in using Outlook e-mail software, as clinical nurses do not use e-mail to communicate in the clinical setting. We received help on how to make folders to organize mail for the two studies. Creating a virtual file cabinet to effectively manage two projects at once improved our ability to keep organized, time-referenced communication.

Lesson 7: Ask for assistance in how to organize electronic research files so that you can efficiently store and access files when needed.

Co-investigators completed the online Collaborative Institutional Training Initiative (CITI) human subject's protection courses and research education training requirements prior to submitting the proposal to the IRB. Proposals were written in stages as a group, and shared electronically with nurse researcher mentors who made suggested wording edits and returned the revised proposal. The back-and-forth sharing was an effective method of proposal development. It allowed us to work independently and, therefore, grow professionally from feedback and changes received from mentors. Essentially, we were able to generate our ideas under the umbrella of doctorate-prepared, experienced nurse researchers. During start-up of proposal writing for the second study, we wrote with more independence, became stronger leads for the study team (which was larger), and had greater confidence in the steps needed to create a research proposal.

Lesson 8: Practice makes perfect; or, since perfection is an illusion, it improves skills and builds confidence.

Tool Selection

Tool selection and implementation were new learning experiences. In order to measure medication adherence we searched the literature for a valid and reliable tool. The instrument the study team desired to use was simple and met requirements based on the research questions. However, before utilizing the tool, we learned there was a fee per study participant. Sample size was 300, and the study was not externally funded, which presented a problem. Team members explored external grant funding, and learned that a minimum requirement to apply was education at a master's degree level, which made the study team ineligible. Co-investigators, with assistance from the hospital librarian, located the owner of the tool at a major university. The professor was contacted, and we requested permission to use the instrument, without charge, in the current study. The professor understood that we would apply for internal funding to cover the costs of use in a follow-up (next phase) intervention study, as needed. Jayne waited in anticipation of the professor's response. Upon receiving the positive e-mail response, the good news was eagerly shared at a nursing council meeting. Trying to maintain composure and professionalism at the podium was difficult when I wanted to shout the team's success far and wide.

Lesson 9: Don't be intimidated by an instrument that requires payment to use, if it is the "best" match with the concept being measured. Ask to use without charge, and you may receive your wish!

Implementation of the medication adherence tool brought an unexpected surprise: following administration, study participants asked how they scored. Upon review of the instrument by the study team, we realized that the scoring legend was typed at the bottom, and that patients may have been answering questions to make us happy, rather than providing accurate responses based on actual adherence. We sought advice from our nurse researcher mentor and chose to remove the scoring legend from the instrument. An amendment to the IRB application was made and approved, and study nurses observed that patients were no longer looking to learn how well they performed, but providing an accurate assessment of adherence.

> *Lesson 10*: Valid and reliable tools can still present with obstacles during use. Pay close attention to data collection for the first 10 cases to determine if revisions are needed.

Proposal Submission to the IRB

The first study was submitted to the IRB with our nurse researcher mentor via phone conference. The website operates in real time, so we were able to view the application from separate locations simultaneously. She provided explanation for each stage in the process and checked the "submit" button when we were ready. The second application was completed by the study team and then reviewed and edited by our nurse researcher mentor. Our confidence level was higher, allowing us to be more independent in leading the process. When it came time to submit the application for the second study, we were excited by our accomplishment. To share our elation, we each put a finger on the mouse, clicked "submit" together, and took a picture to send via text message to a team member who could not be present for the memorable event.

> *Lesson 11*: "Doing," rather than observing or receiving didactic education, builds confidence in the processes of research initiation.

DIGGING INTO DATA COLLECTION AND ANALYSIS

Database Development

When it was time to create a database for both studies, study teams learned that REDCap (an online research database from Vanderbilt University) was available to all Cleveland Clinic hospital organization employees. A nurse from the office where the medication-adherence study was taking place suggested using REDCap; our nurse researcher mentor agreed, so that became the plan. Tutorials were available to assist with database set up; however, nurses on the study team found them to be intimidating. We requested assistance from our nurse researcher mentor, who helped set up via phone conference. We later noted that one of our forms was inadvertently missing, and were able to create the form in REDCap from skills learned.

We were curious about different databases available. The IBM Statistical Package for Social Science (SPSS) Statistics database was purchased specifically for our nursing research program and was available on one computer within the hospital. Logistically, it was practical to collect data and enter it into a database within the hospital. The BP database was developed with guidance from our nurse researcher mentor. We also received guidelines for data entry that were used for graduate students who would input data when we were ready.

A secure place to store and access research files was needed. As clinical nurses, we did not have access to locking file cabinets. Data collection was initiated without a specific plan for data storage, despite requests to nurse leadership. In one request, we included the chief nursing officer in the e-mail request. As a temporary solution, a file cabinet was provided in the nurse manager's office. A research cabinet was secured. Obtaining keys for co-investigators and students involved in the research study took time, and required us to change our initial plan, as we had to limit data collectors based on the number of keys available. The chief nursing officer later provided a secure, central file storage location for use by all nurses participating in research.

> *Lesson 12*: Learn to be flexible and, when flexibility is not an option due to human subjects protection, be ready to flex plans.

As clinical nurses and research nurses, we felt we were impacting peers through our excitement about being involved in research. The BP study was the first research led by nurses in critical care. As we discussed our study, critical care nurses were acknowledged for their data collection contribution to nursing practice. Through interactions with nurses that revolved around research, other nurses started conversations about research. We became members of the hospital shared governance nursing research council and raised the topic of research in Nursing Congress (a nursing council to which all other councils report). Further, Jayne became a member of the Nursing Institute Research Council, which serves the entire health care system and provides an opportunity for her to share her spirit of inquiry.

Data Collection and Cleaning

For float nurses, change is synonymous with an average work day; however, adding research to the mix took the term "float" to a new level. The first study took us to an outpatient office, which was unfamiliar territory. Comparatively, it would be like visiting a foreign country, where things were unfamiliar and the welcome mat was not always rolled out. We were excited about what we were doing in getting answers to research questions on medication adherence, but unsure about how to start the process of data collection, including what specifically to say to potential subjects. Our clinical experiences and general nursing backgrounds did not match the skill set needed to approach this new endeavor. By now, we knew our next step: Ask our mentor for guidance. The research quality coordinator (a non-nurse whose main role is to oversee and monitor the quality of nurse-led research in the nursing research program) was consulted and provided a role-play opportunity with scripting. Then, we put aside our apprehensions and jumped into data collection, as planned.

Lesson 13: When clinical nurses are conducting research, they need to be ready to step outside their comfort zone.

Despite preparation for data collection, unexpected challenges arose. To foster a positive working relationship with the staff of the ambulatory office on the first day of data collection, we brought fresh cinnamon rolls with a thank you note of appreciation for sharing space and patients with the research study team. We also offered to meet privately if concerns or problems were raised. The office had a research nurse who supported physician-led research. We were able to share her file space and initiate general research-based communications. She approached us regarding a need to document study enrollment in subjects' medical records. We were not trained in recording research participation in patients' records. We showed her an IRB resource that indicated that our study was low risk and did not require the documentation she requested, which was confirmed by our nurse researcher mentor. Our mentor described different levels of risk in research, and explained that our research was led by nurses and independent of physician oversight. In the process of being questioned by an established research nurse, our emotions shifted from feeling apprehensive to feeling empowered and proud of our accomplishments.

Lesson 14: Like many things in life, research comes in many forms and levels of risk; each has its own guidelines and rules of conduct.

The spatial constraints of the office posed a new challenge. A nurse practitioner's (NP) office was provided for our use when not occupied. On the first day, all co-investigators were present to ensure high internal consistency in data collection. Due to an unusually high patient volume, the NP was called in (an unexpected event to our plans) and work space reassignment was necessary. The cardiology group manages a high volume of patients and the team functioned like a well-oiled machine, with everyone knowing their roles and the flow of activities. Although we had the best intentions, our presence disrupted the flow of a very efficient system. The alternate work space we were assigned encroached upon their ability to complete work smoothly. As a result, we were abrasively approached by one physician, with his staff present, and instructed to limit study nurses to one-per-day. He must have missed the cinnamon rolls and the note accompanying them. We were so excited to finally get started, and then felt deflated by multiple obstacles, including the manner in which the physician approached us. As new researchers, we were not prepared to deal with the extraneous obstacles we encountered. When we discussed the events with our nurse researcher mentor, she was reassuring in her response that this was not an uncommon occurrence. The limitations imposed on us to only have one study nurse in the office per day decreased data collection and altered our time line. Reluctantly, Jayne initiated contact with the physician by e-mail, and he relented on only allowing one person per day, with conditions. It took strength, courage, and support from our nurse researcher mentor to return to the office to collect data, but it also led to a new resource. We forged new relationships with office nurses, who were willing to have us there on high-volume days, providing an opportunity to enhance data collection.

Lesson 12 Revisited: Learn to be flexible, and, when flexibility is not an option, learn to flex plans.

The BP study was conducted in familiar surroundings, but there were obstacles in data collection as well. We attended shared governance and staff meetings to elicit support and inform staff. A study announcement was created and distributed to mailboxes, posted in units, and e-mailed to nurse managers. Designated unit and float pool nurses were recruited and trained as experts to standardize the data collection procedure and engage nurses. Unit nurses were mixed regarding their desire to participate in data collection, as study involvement required taking extra BPs and recording results on a case report form. Since research was new to unit nurses, its value was not recognized. We requested leadership support to encourage nurses' participation in data collection, monitored completed case report forms for accuracy, and re-educated nurses on proper procedure, as needed. Originally, each study team member was assigned to monitor one ICU for the number of completed data collection forms and accuracy of content. As team members had unanticipated absences, we took over the process fully, and found that we enjoyed the process immensely. As a suggestion from our nurse researcher mentor, graphs were routinely posted in each ICU to show progress toward subject enrollment goals, and indirectly to keep nurses engaged, compare unit participation levels, and provide incentive (healthy competition) among units (see Figure 11.1). Creating the bar graphs and best-practice flyer provided another learning opportunity. They were displayed on the professional practice model boards in each unit, so study progress could be shared in daily huddles. Graphs included data collection best practices to encourage proper case report form documentation. Nurses and office staff who were especially supportive during the data collection phase received notes of appreciation from us.

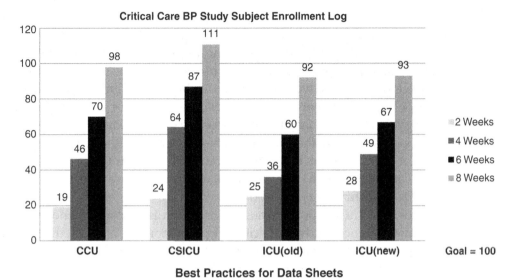

FIGURE 11.1 Sample enrollment update provided to nurses during data collection.

Note: ICU (old) and ICU (new) units treat mixed medical-surgical patients.

BP, blood pressure; CCU, coronary care unit; CSICU, cardiothoracic surgical intensive care unit; IRB, institutional review board.

Strategies utilized to encourage nurses to provide documentation of usual care data on the case report form were at the suggestion of our nurse researcher mentor.

Lesson 15: Staff engagement is vital for successful data collection procedures.

Data collection takes time, and since this phase was completed on a parallel time line for both studies, we alternated between them, based on ambulatory office volume. We worked within our budgeted allotment of hours, which was initially 4 hours per week per nurse.

Over time we navigated through two studies concomitantly, balancing our time between data collection (the BP study) and data query resolution (the medication adherence study). In the BP study, unit nurses completed usual-care data collection, reducing the amount of time spent in completing case report forms; however, forms were monitored by us for completeness and medical record review data were collected.

When recruitment was slow in the office, we used the time to update leadership on their data query findings that required follow up, and enter data into the database. It was good to have another study to focus on that generated excitement and support, rather than initial resistance. Timelines for the studies were parallel. We worked within our budgetary limitations, at first being given 4-hour increments each week to collect data. We re-evaluated our work strategy each week to facilitate maintenance of the medication adherence study time line, as we were the primary data collectors. We had to request additional time for data collection to reach the predetermined sample size. As we became more comfortable with data collection, we became more efficient in the process.

Data cleaning was not laborious when we collected and input data, since we monitored case report forms and instruments for completeness in the medication adherence study. Data cleaning was more involved in the BP study as multiple nurses took part in obtaining BPs and providing results on case report forms. To ensure Charlson comorbidity index sheets matched BP cases, we used the back side of case report forms. This allowed us the opportunity to practice environmentally and cost-conscious behaviors. Data collection also included data pulls from administrative databases. Although an analyst provided data, we were called upon by our biostatisticians to provide missing data or review erroneous data. Although data cleaning took time, it was rewarding to contribute to this process, and it opened our eyes to the careful attention given to ensuring data were accurate and complete.

Understanding Analyses and Disseminating Findings

In the medication adherence study, results were shared with co-investigators by the nurse researcher mentor. Despite repeated explanations given, nurses had difficulty interpreting data analyses. The language and methods of analysis were complex and not easily understood by untrained nurses. We feel that nurses need to learn how to interpret findings from publications (and research analysis reports) by becoming familiar with statistical terms. Statistical analysis methods were foreign and challenged nurses despite their participation in research.

In the BP study, the process of data interpretation continued to challenge us. There was a staggering amount of statistical data presented to us. Additionally, the entire team was unable to meet to review findings when initially presented; team understanding was a little like Swiss cheese, with a lot of holes. Our nurse researcher mentor attempted to coach us to identify significant study findings, only to find we still needed her expertise and guidance. This is something that we find perplexing. We are not dim, we are professionals, but we wonder: Will we ever get it? On a positive note, we learned about the relationship between statistical and clinical significance. Overall, we understand statistical significance, based on the p value, but not necessarily how to express the analysis in written words.

Dissemination of findings is an expectation; communicating research findings accurately and intelligently, for acceptance in a respected peer-reviewed journal can be challenging. Not long into the process, we realized research has its own verbiage and we encountered a language barrier. Learning the language of research is essential to interpreting findings, as well as developing a proposal, and finally disseminating one's own findings in a meaningful way that other researchers will respect. In preparation for this step, we have become comfortable using the term "manuscript" and use it fluently. This particular term has prompted us to take pause when our fellow nurses ask what we mean when we refer to it in conversation. In respect to dissemination of our research, we found ourselves at a new roadblock. We attended workshops on writing for publication and went back to our nurse researcher mentors for direction. We learned about an impact factor and how to choose a peer-reviewed journal for publication. Templates were extracted from our nursing research program website to provide guidance. Time was scheduled to write that was convenient for co-investigators. With advice of our nurse researcher mentors, appropriate journals were selected for both studies. Currently, both studies are in the dissemination phase; both will be presented at an upcoming nursing research conference and the medication adherence study is being developed into a manuscript.

THE BIG PICTURE IN NURSING RESEARCH

Mentorship Versus Independent Work

As novice research nurses, we were not aware of the many research processes or time commitments needed when we embarked on this new experience. Nurse researcher mentors shared research process steps as we were ready, but there was no global explanation at the onset. For some nurses, it may be overwhelming to have advance knowledge of the complete process, but it proved to be a favorable experience for us. In total, the research procedure was extensive, but was divided into concise steps, and from our perspective, was manageable.

In our nursing research program, doctorate-prepared nurse researchers mentor nurses based on subject, expertise, and patient population of proposed studies. This was true of the latter of our projects, not the former. In the medication adherence study, we specifically asked a nurse researcher mentor who was present at the workshop to guide us, as we had met her previously and she had assisted us in formulating research questions. For the BP study, it was a little more intimidating, yet exciting, as the nursing research program department head, based on her area of expertise, offered mentorship. She attended our initial meeting where interest in the study was explored. Research was not commonplace for clinical nurses at our hospital at the time. Having the department head support our research idea was a big deal. Her credentials take up a line by themselves, and we speculated she would be too busy with leadership work to attend a meeting with us, regular clinical nurses. We believe her presence added to the excitement of this research project and was the fuel that ignited and maintained the forward momentum of the study.

We were nurtured by our first mentor through all the research processes. Our mentor was like the kindergarten teacher everyone wants when they leave the comfort of home. We learned from her that there were no potholes we could not maneuver around. We would e-mail her when something unusual came up, and she would provide a solution. When we progressed to the second study, we had learned enough to function more independently, and thus required less direct supervision. We had left the crawling and learning stage to the stand stage of research, and were now ready to take steps and practice running. Knowing the department head had other responsibilities, we not only wanted to please her, we also did not want to burden her with simple research processes that we knew we could handle on our own.

> *Lesson 16*: Analysis and mentorship by expert nurse researchers may feel like you are taking a foreign language course. Repetition in learning is crucial. Novice research nurses must speak up—ask for explanations and practice teach-back to ensure you understand your data analyses accurately.

Making Time

Throughout the research experience, we recognized that setting aside time was one of the most valuable ingredients to success. To contribute to new knowledge, nurses need to set aside specific time from usual clinical duties to participate in research activities including literature review, proposal development, data collection, database set up and input, data cleaning, understanding analysis, and dissemination. Clinical research, even when clinical nurses participate, requires an ongoing time commitment from the research study team and nurse leadership. Nurse managers must be willing to allocate time to complete research work. It may be important to discuss time management up front so that clinical nurses and management can assist in a successful research experience.

> *Lesson 17*: Be ready to set aside ample time for research process work, as time is an essential component for success in research.

In summary, we found that our first attempts at research provided a menagerie of learning experiences. The experience provided opportunities to learn the processes of research and how they advance the foundation of nursing practice. Providing the highest level of patient care is dependent on nursing research and evidence-based nursing practices. It is our hope that novice research nurses will benefit from our lessons learned and experiences, and that nursing leadership will recognize that mentorship by expert nurse researchers is critical to success. Mentorship takes time, and often the work of the mentor is really to be a coach, to demonstrate and observe return demonstrations by novice research nurses. Mentorship in nursing research aids clinical nurses to make the transition to a higher level of clinical practice and develops a spirit of inquiry that is so important in our ever-changing field of patient-centered health care.

Acknowledgment

We would like to respectfully acknowledge our nurse leadership at Hillcrest Hospital and nurse researcher mentors for their support in our research. It has been a remarkable journey.

STORIES FROM THE FIELD
Mary Beth Modic

The statement "curiosity is more important than knowledge" is attributed to one of the greatest thinkers and most prolific researchers of the 20th century, Albert Einstein. Curiosity is an essential attribute of a researcher. It compels us to be open to possibilities, question patterns and relationships, and test hunches. It directs our care, our education, and further research.

Many nurses embrace using nursing research but feel unprepared to carry out a research study on their own. Often-cited barriers include lack of time, resources, or skill. Although these certainly can be obstacles, it is important to remember that nursing is a relatively young profession and needs research to guide and influence its practice. Even if the results are not statistically significant, all rigorous studies contribute to nursing science.

This section describes several research studies that I (MBM) conducted and offer lessons learned from a novice researcher.

Lessons Learned

1. Say "yes" to nursing research opportunities.
2. Begin with a small study.
3. Anticipate that your study will take twice as long as you planned.

4. Use technology.
5. Participate in a qualitative study.
6. Investigate a "sacred cow."
7. Publish your results.

LESSONS 1 AND 2: SAY "YES" TO NURSING RESEARCH OPPORTUNITIES AND BEGIN SMALL

The first lesson learned is to say "yes" to research opportunities. Pursue opportunities to engage in research studies, if not at your own organization, then at a college or university near your home or place of employment. Seek out a research mentor. This individual can help demystify the research process. Participate in a journal club, either virtually or in person. Reading and reviewing current research publications will help you gain knowledge in evaluating research for rigor and quality.

Lesson two addresses the breadth and depth of your research study. Your first study should be small in scope so that it is manageable. My first research study examined the knowledge of nurses working on cardiology and cardiovascular surgical units and their mastery of diabetes survival skills. It was a 20-item questionnaire that addressed knowledge of diet, oral medications, hypoglycemia rescue, and insulin administration. Nurses were asked to identify whether the statement was true or false and whether they had a need for more information. The survey also queried nurses' comfort in teaching survival skills. Ninety registered nurses completed the survey. In analysis, data revealed that nurses' knowledge and comfort relating to diabetes survival skills were low. Additionally, in 35% of the total items, there was a significant association between need for more knowledge and incorrect responses (Modic et al., 2009).

Data collection was completed in approximately 6 weeks. The most time consuming aspect of the study was entering data into a database, followed by determining content validity of the survey. The entire study process, from designing the research question to interpreting results, took 18 months to complete. Another 6 months were spent writing and submitting the manuscript.

LESSON 3: ANTICIPATE THAT A RESEARCH STUDY WILL TAKE LONGER TO COMPLETE THAN EXPECTED

The third lesson addresses the issue of time. Often, a research study may require more time than was initially anticipated. This was true of my second study, which was an observational study. I was curious to learn how well patients with diabetes and receiving insulin ate in the hospital. I also wanted to know what food items patients were eating off from their meal trays. A convenience sample of patients from two medical and two surgical units were recruited for the study. The study required that an investigator observe what was consumed from the meal tray. The food items were compared with the items that appeared on the meal ticket. Patients were interviewed if meal consumption was less than 100%.

In preparation for the study, each investigator was observed by two dietitians until concordance of meal consumption was achieved. The practice period took 2 weeks. Four investigators were assigned to collect data during the week and two investigators collected data on weekends. Data collection spanned 5 months. A total of 2,945 meal trays were observed from 434 patients.

Patients were enrolled in the study at the time of their admission and data were collected beginning with their first lunch meal for 4 consecutive days. A chart review provided data on patient demographics, weight, and prescribed diet. Dietitians calculated the caloric and macronutrient needs for each patient. Data were entered into the database immediately after collection to minimize entry errors and fatigue. In analysis, we learned that patients ate 37% to 39% of calculated caloric needs and 43% to 47% of their carbohydrate recommendations. Low carbohydrate consumption has significant implications for prandial insulin administration (Modic et al., 2011). The results reinforced the findings of previous researchers that meal consumption by hospitalized patients was inadequate, and that caloric and protein intake does not meet the daily recommended requirements.

The study took 2 years to complete. Data needed to be "cleaned" for accuracy and analyzed. It took another 2 years to write the manuscript. Observational research studies can be labor intensive, but a well-designed study can yield important findings.

When I first embarked on this research with my nutrition colleagues, I had no idea the study would take so long to complete. The study required additional work hours for each investigator as evening meals and weekend observations were beyond the standard workdays and work hours. In addition, most of the writing of the manuscript occurred during evening hours or on weekends. However, the research team was committed to seeing the study through to the end. We knew it was important to disseminate our findings and that we had important findings to share. We shared a passion for the topic and were invigorated with our findings. We were re-inspired to keep writing as we added each new paragraph to our manuscript.

Nutrition in the critically ill receives a great deal of attention in the nursing literature. The same has not been true for patients on medical surgical units until recently. Many hospitals implemented a "room service" program, similar to hotels, to address missed meals and make food available when patients wish to eat (Mohd Nor, 2010). Our study findings support this national nutrition initiative as one solution to inadequate meal consumption in the hospital.

LESSON 4: USE TECHNOLOGY

Another important lesson learned is to use available technology whenever possible. Seek out possibilities to collect data electronically. Surveys can be designed so that participants must completely respond to the previous question before proceeding to the next question, preventing incomplete or missing data.

My next study investigated nurses' knowledge of inpatient diabetes management principles. Level of knowledge was assessed using a 20-item pretest prior to a 4-hour diabetes course and retesting immediately after the course. The sample consisted of 2,250 registered nurses. All specialties except neonatal and operating room nurses were represented. Although knowledge increased, as reflected by improvement in posttest scores, knowledge gaps related to insulin remained. Moreover, nurses had high levels of comfort and familiarity and low levels of knowledge (Modic et al., 2014b).

The nurses' knowledge study took a very long time to complete because nurses answered the pre- and posttest on paper. This meant that there were 4,500 tests to score and enter into the IBM SPSS database! I never considered using Scantron™ sheets (in which responses on sheets are faxed directly into a database, similar to a voting booth) for the participants to complete or employing an audience participation system to capture their answers. The challenge in data collection resulted from my lack of awareness of technology that could have expedited the work.

As a result of the nurses' knowledge-study results, several resources were developed to assist nurses with inpatient diabetes management. THINK-CARDS,™ laminated pocket cards that contain information about insulin therapeutics, oral glucose lowering agents, insulin pump and IV insulin infusion management, and survival skill content, were created. A diabetes education website that houses information such as a carbohydrate counting guide, diabetes patient education handouts, current evidence-based practice literature, and frequently asked questions (FAQs) was designed to provide "just in time" answers. A diabetes management mentor program, a unit-based diabetes resource nurse program, was also initiated to assist bedside nurses with solving problems, providing accurate diabetes survival skill education, and identifying patients at risk for hypoglycemia.

LESSON 5: QUALITATIVE RESEARCH WILL ENRICH NEW KNOWLEDGE LEARNED

The fifth lesson learned was to participate in a qualitative study if you have the chance. Qualitative research captures how people experience a given research topic. It enriches the knowledge collected in a study by encouraging participants to share their stories, opinions, beliefs, and emotions. When coupled with quantitative research, qualitative research can help interpret the results obtained in a quantitative study.

A study that I recently completed was a mixed-methods design. I studied caring behaviors and perceptions of nurses and patients hospitalized with diabetes. I was interested in this topic because effective diabetes management requires highly knowledgeable and empowered patients. Conversely, patients with diabetes are often labeled "noncompliant" when their blood glucose values are "out of control" or they are "not following their diet." I wanted to learn what nurses thought were effective caring behaviors that they used with patients who have diabetes. I also wanted to hear what caring behaviors patients with diabetes reported receiving from clinical nurses.

In this study, nurses reported teaching, listening, and supporting as caring behaviors, with teaching being the most cited behavior by 76% of nurses. One nurse recounted her diabetic teaching this way, *"I find out what patients know about their diabetes and I learn from those that know themselves well."* Another nurse shared this comment *"I assess my patient's level of knowledge regarding her diabetes, determining what she does at home and how well it works for her"* (Modic, Siedlecki, Quinn-Griffin, & Fitzpatrick, 2014a). Statements suggested that nurses believed that learning is reciprocal and that getting to know patients is important to delivering patient-centered care.

Patients in the caring behaviors study identified (a) provided information completed, (b) surveillance/monitoring, and (c) listened to their concerns as reflective of caring behaviors. Interestingly, none of the patients reported receiving formal education from nurses. Rather, they received updates about activities for the day or results of blood point-of-care glucose tests. Many patients described the importance of being heard. One patient expressed his sentiment this way, *"Since I am blind, I get a sense of how caring a nurse is going to be by the tone of her voice and how quickly she speaks to me. . . . I know nurses are busy, but in the truly caring nurses, you never hear that they are rushed in their voice or in their footsteps as they walk away"* (Modic et al., 2014a).

As a result of this study, the diabetes education website added content on communication techniques that can be used to convey empathy, active listening, and eliciting patient concerns. Links to evidence-based literature that explores the concepts of adherence, motivational interviewing, and relationship-centered care were added to the website.

LESSON 6: SACRED COW CAMPAIGN

Deciding what to study can be challenging as the world of nursing is so broad and ever expanding. My sixth lesson learned is that investigating a "sacred cow" can be an interesting journey into the world of nursing research.

A sacred cow is an outdated practice that has been proven ineffective, costly, or unnecessary. Practices have been passed on from one generation of nurses to another without evidence to support their use (Makic,VonRueden, Rauen, & Chadwick, 2011). My interest in safe insulin administration practices stemmed from my previous research in which we identified that nurses' knowledge of insulin therapeutics was not optimal. The double insulin checking study was developed to determine whether a well-delineated double checking procedure was effective in preventing insulin administration errors. While the practice has been recommended by The Joint Commission and the Institute of Safe Medication Practices (ISMP); there is no clinical research evidence to support its use.

LESSON 7: PUBLISHING RESULTS IS CRITICAL TO ADVANCING SCIENCE

The final lesson learned is that publishing your findings is critical to dissemination. A podium or poster presentation, although important, is not sufficient. Publishing your research allows other researchers to critique your study and replicate or refute your findings. It also serves as a way to establish ownership of an idea or process. Publishing is also time consuming, and oftentimes comes with rejection, rewriting or revising, and resubmitting.

   After facilitating the diabetes management mentor program for 3 years, I was curious about the impact the program had on individual nurses who participated. I was interested in learning about nurses' perceptions of important differences they make in mentoring other nurses on their units to enhance knowledge, skill, and confidence in diabetes management. Seventeen diabetes management mentors on 11 different nursing units were interviewed regarding their contributions. Mentors who participated in this study spoke clearly and passionately about their role. Three themes emerged as mentors described their experiences: professional courage, role modeling confidence, and making a difference (Modic, Sorrell, Sauvey, Modic, & Hancock, 2015). One nurse remarked:

> Sometimes it's the nurse's knowledge base, sometimes like newer nurses—they're not sure whether they should give the insulin or not. . . . I'm thinking about a patient on an insulin pump who came from home with it and the nurse had never seen it before and didn't know what to do, and I kind of guided her through the process, and, you know, we just started at square one. And then we went to the resource on the intranet, we went to the policy. The policy spells it out really clearly what you need to do . . . There are a lot of details to that—so that was a real positive experience because the nurse felt, you know, confident that she could do it on her own the next time.

Another nurse shared this thought with the interviewer:

> I see myself differently. The role allows me to sort of be an educator to other nurses. It provides some type of "officiality" or positional authority where people expect you to know some answers—and hopefully you will! [laughs] . . . It's offered me opportunities I wouldn't have had otherwise.

The research paper was rejected by several journals until my coauthors and I changed the focus and rewrote a significant portion. We believed that we had evidence that supported a diabetes management mentor program as best practice. Mentors spoke about their influence on inpatient diabetes care and also described its impact on their professional development. We hope study findings will encourage others to replicate the research methods it uses so that the passion and commitment bedside nurses have for their work can be promoted.

In summary, nursing research is an important endeavor. It is simultaneously challenging and invigorating, time consuming and gratifying, tedious and liberating. My advice to you, the reader and future researcher, is: Be curious! Ask questions! Get going!

REFERENCES

Makic, M. B., VonRueden, K. T., Rauen, C. A., & Chadwick, J. (2011). Evidence-based practice habits: Putting more sacred cows out to pasture. *Critical Care Nurse, 31*(2), 38–61.

Modic, M. B., Albert, N., Nutter, B., Coughlin, R., Murray, T., Spence, J., & Broscovich, D. (2009). Diabetes teaching is not for the faint of heart: Are cardiac nurses up to the challenge? *Journal of Cardiovascular Nursing, 24*(6), 439–446.

Modic, M. B., Kozak, A., Siedlecki, S., Nowak, D., Parella, D., Morris, M. P., . . . Binon, S. (2011). Do we know what our patients with diabetes are eating in the hospital? *Diabetes Spectrum, 24*(2), 100–106.

Modic, M. B., Siedlecki, S. L., Quinn-Griffin, M., & Fitzpatrick, J. J. (2014a). Caring behaviors: Perceptions of acute care nurses and hospitalized patients with diabetes. *Journal of Patient Experience, 1*(1), 26–30.

Modic, M. B., Sorrell, J., Sauvey, R., Modic, J., & Hancock, K. K. (2015). Creating expertise in inpatient diabetes care: A diabetes management mentor program. *Journal of Nursing Care Quality, 30*(1), 12–16.

Modic, M. B., Vanderbilt, A., Siedlecki, S. L., Sauvey, R., Kaser, N., & Yager, C. (2014b). Diabetes management unawareness: What do bedside nurses know? *Applied Nursing Research, 27*(3), 157–161.

Mohd Nor, Z. (2010). *Hospital foodservice directors identify the important aspects when implementing room service in hospital foodservice.* (Unpublished master's thesis). Iowa State University, Ames, Iowa.

INDEX

Printed in the United States
By Bookmasters